WATER BIRTH
WISDOM

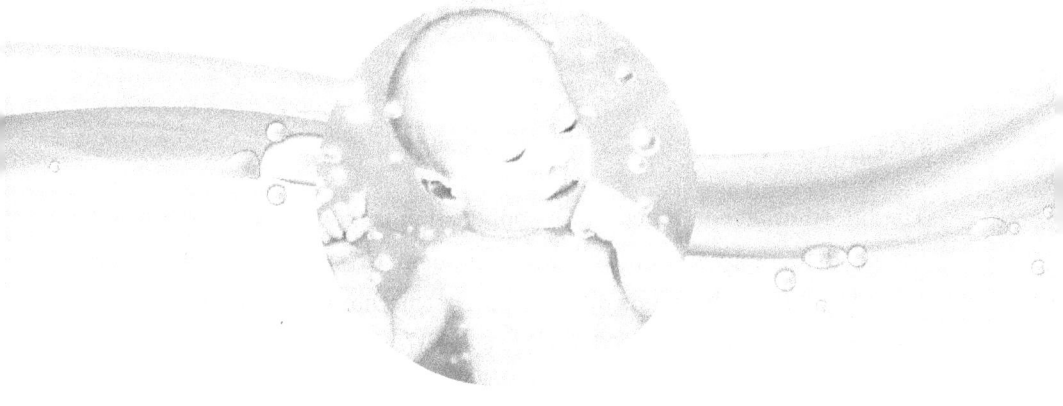

Rima Star

Praeclarus Press, LLC
©2022 Rima Star.

www.PraeclarusPress.com

Praeclarus Press, LLC 2504 Sweetgum Lane
Amarillo, Texas 79124 USA 806-367-9950

www.PraeclarusPress.com

DISCLAIMER

The information contained in this publication is advisory only and is not intended to replace sound clinical judgment or individualized patient care. The author disclaims all warranties, whether expressed or implied, including any warranty as the quality, accuracy, safety, or suitability of this information for any particular purpose.

ISBN: 978-1-946665-53-9

Cover Design: Ken Tackett

Developmental Editing: Kathleen Kendall-Tackett

Copyediting: Chris Tackett

Layout & Design: Nelly Murariu

*I dedicate this book to
my three wonderful children,
all born in water:
Mela, Orien, and Hank.*

CONTENTS

Chapter 3. Water Delivery 127

Chapter 4. Water and Bonding

Figures

Figure 1.1. Peyton playing "poke" with her brother.

Figure 1.2. Peyton's delight at being poked back.

Figure 2.1. My daughter Orien laboring in privacy with the support of two trusted people – her husband Andy and her midwife.

Figure 2.2. A couple takes a nature walk during early labor.

Figure 2.3. My daughter Orien and her husband Andy on a nature walk in early labor.

Figure 2.4. Technology at the service of the birthing couple. But where is the technology? It is, of course, this highly sophisticated jacuzzi, the maze of pipes that bring the water, and the electricity that warms that water. Technologies that are truly supportive of birth tend to recede into the background and go unnoticed, while the laboring woman is in the foreground.

Figure 2.5. Robbie as "Eve in Eden" in "laborland" in her hot tub.

Figure 2.6. Robbie in the tub in heavy, active labor, using her husband's arms to pull against and with her 4-year-old daughter Peyton watching.

Figure 2.7. Robbie about to give birth in bed. As her birth facilitator/doula, I was on the other side of the bed, allowing the midwives, Cathy and Debbie, space to deal with the brief shoulder dystocia her baby experienced. Yes, upright positions for birth are best, but when you have been up and moving around a lot during labor, it does not matter if you lie down for the moments of birth, and side-lying is better than on your back, as it allows more pelvic space. Note the oxygen mask Robbie's husband Robert is holding over her face at the midwives' suggestion.

She found that to be an extremely empowering use of technology, as the pure oxygen gave her added energy just when she needed it most.

Figure 2.8. The baby's head is out, and Robbie cradles it in her hand. She said, "That feeling is forever imprinted in my hand's palm and my heart's memory."

Figure 2.9. Robbie silently asking Jason what he needed.

Figure 2.10. Baby Jason mellows out in his tub.

Figure 2.11. Robbie birthing Jason with Peyton (right) and Mela (left) watching. At one point, Peyton dragged in a high barstool so she could sit on it and have a better view.

Figure 2.12. Peyton sitting on her barstool, clutching a boy doll—for Robbie had intuitively known the baby would be a boy—with Mela about to climb up to join her.

Figure 2.13. The newborn family, as Peyton approaches to meet her new brother. But first, she had taken a good look at Robbie's vagina, as, even though she had watched the whole birth, she was still astonished that something so big could come through something so small.

Figures 3.1. and 3.2. My daughter Orien in "laborland" with her husband Andy in their inflatable tub, which they placed in their bedroom close to their bed and filled with a hose that they ran from a heater.

Figure 3.3. A birthing tub in a New Zealand birth center with vinyl cushions for the midwives to sit or kneel on.

Figure 3.4. Pulling up a mobile stool on wheels for the midwife to sit by the edge of the tub in another New Zealand birth center.

Figure 3.5. Orien's two midwives check the fetal heart rate with a Doppler.

Foreword

Almost 40 years ago, in 1984, Rima Star was my doula for my son Jason's home birth, though she prefers the term "birth facilitator," which to her means not only helping women prepare for and give birth, but also helping anyone to process their birth experience – to remember their birth and to heal any resultant traumas. Although Rima trained as a midwife, she chose the career of birth facilitator instead so that she could serve more people. Rima is one of the best-known rebirthers/breath therapists in the United States – she has an amazing talent for using a combination of connected breathing and massage to put her clients into an altered state of consciousness, during which they can re-experience any traumas, from those that may have happened in their own births on throughout their lives, express, and heal them in the safe context of Rima's space and the loving energy she holds.

Rima labored and gave birth to all three of her children—Mela, Orien, and Hank—in water; you can read about those births in her first book, *The Healing Power of Birth* (1986), so-named by the world-famous obstetrician Michel Odent, one of the pioneers of water labor and water birth. That book is difficult to obtain on Amazon and other sites, but Rima herself has a number of copies, and you can order them directly from her at rimabethstar@gmail.com. Over the years, she has traveled widely, including to the former Soviet Union, to give talks, workshops, and to attend people's births. She has appeared on many TV shows as well, bringing her youngest child with her and breastfeeding on television as needed. One of her TV interviews was with an obstetrician who was vehemently opposed to home birth and had written a book contravening water birth, but during the show, he ended up asking Rima many questions, and at the end, he stood up, faced the audience, and said, "If you are like Ms. Star, great, have a home birth and a water birth with a midwife – and otherwise come to the hospital and we will take care of you." In other words, he completely changed his opinion after listening to Rima's answers to his questions.

Rima is one of the wisest, most loving people I know, and so this present book, *Water Birth Wisdom*, is aptly named, as it is full of the wisdom and knowledge about the use of water during pregnancy, labor, and birth that she has gained over many years of experience facilitating hundreds of women and couples to prepare for and then to labor and/or birth in water. The pages of this book are full, not only of her water birth wisdom, but also of actual stories of those who have used the healing, gravity-relieving medium of water during pregnancy, labor, birth, and the postpartum period. Rima calls this water medium "liquid love." She has also included imaginary stories in each chapter written from what she envisions the baby's experience to be like.

This book almost didn't happen! Rima wrote it years ago, and then life took over, and she only recently rediscovered it on her computer. It has been my pleasure to help her update the references to make this book as contemporary as possible.

This magical book will show you how to both exercise and be playful in the water during pregnancy, how to plan and prepare for a water labor and/or birth, and how to stay in or enter your tub for postpartum bonding. Rima gets specific about what sort of tubs work best, what kind of water to use, what to put in it or not, and what temperature the water should be. If you are wanting to use water for any phase of the perinatal period or thinking about that as a possibility, then this is the book for you! This book is also relevant to and supportive of all birth professionals, to include in and enrich their understandings and practices.

And it is about so much more than the use of water! Rima also carefully and lyrically explains the processes of conception, the growth of the fetus, the multiple ways in which birth can occur, the importance of the birth environment, and how pregnant people and their partners can best prepare themselves physically, emotionally, psychologically, and spiritually for labor, birth, the post-partum period, and parenting. She describes birth as art, as the weaving of a beautiful tapestry in which all present are essential threads. She stresses that the baby is a conscious being from conception on, and the possibilities for and the importance of mother-baby communication, both in the womb and out. Far from insisting on water labor and birth, she emphasizes that parents should follow their intuitions and any messages they receive from their baby about where and how the birth should take place, noting that plans can change in the moment, as birth is ever-surprising. The many possibilities she presents for both home and hospital births, and her visions for a more enlightened future for birth, will open her readers' minds to ideas they likely would not have thought of had they not read this inspiring book!

Robbie Davis-Floyd, PhD

Adjunct Professor, Department of Anthropology,
Rice University, Houston, Texas

Author of *Birth as an American Rite of Passage* (1992, 2003, 2022)

Chapter 1

WATER AND PREGNANCY

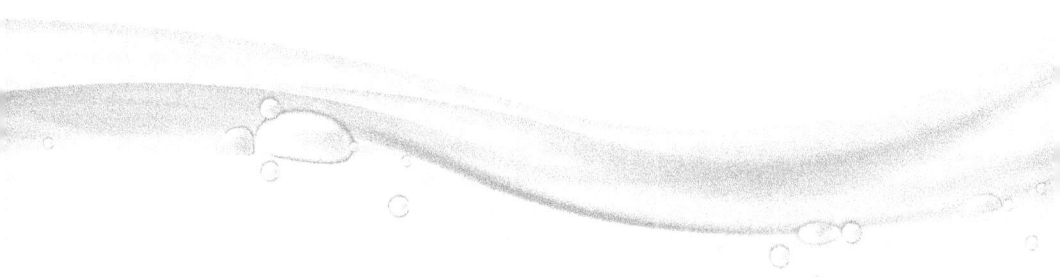

Evolutionarily speaking, we humans are curious creatures. We have much in common not only with higher primates like chimpanzees—with whom we share 98% of our genes—but also with sea mammals. In fact, the "aquatic ape theory" postulates that humans have more in common with sea mammals than with land mammals, and that there was, indeed, a timespan of many millions of years when some higher primates adapted to living in the oceans before they once again came back onto the land as their primary habitat As Elaine Morgan states in her book *The Aquatic Ape*:

> Among mammals, the first to return to the water, some 70 million years ago, were the cetaceans—whales, dolphins and porpoises. Like all mammals they are warm-blooded, breathe air, give birth to live offspring, and suckle their young ... The next to go into the sea, more than 50 million years ago, were vegetarian hoofed mammals related to the elephant. Their descendants are the sirenians, or sea cows ... Between 25-30 million years ago some bearlike carnivorous mammals took to the water. These were the ancestors of the present-day

fur seals, sea lions and walruses ... The aquatic theory
envisages that during this period one group of apes
embarked on a distinct path of evolution by adapting
to an aquatic environment—just as other species had
done earlier. Later, when the waters receded and new
ecological opportunities opened up, they returned to
their former terrestrial lifestyle. But they brought with
them a package of inbuilt aquatic adaptations, which
they still demonstrably retain.[1]

This theory appears to answer many of the questions about why
humans are so different from other higher primates. It may also
be an evolutionary explanation about the friendly and unique
relationships between cetaceans (whales and dolphins) and
humans. These relationships are evidenced in the mythologies
of many cultures, and certainly in the current interest in communication with dolphins.[2]

The possibility that our ancestors spent millions of years
swimming as aquatic apes in the waters of Mother Ocean is an
interesting one to ponder. Some of the ways humans differ from
other higher primates include being hairless, the location of fat
immediately under the skin, perspiration, weeping, walking
erect, and face-to-face copulation.[3] These characteristics are
shared with aquatic mammals. Elaine Morgan attributes these
changes to convergent evolution: "the process by which animals
of quite separate origins grow to resemble one another when
they adopt the same habitat or lifestyle."[4] Perhaps this genetic
memory has something to do with predisposing women to seek
out the sound and experience of water, particularly during their
pregnancies. Having your own small ocean inside of you with a
small "aquatic ape" swimming within may stimulate an ancient
memory of a time in our evolutionary cycle when we freely swam

and moved within the oceans of the earth. Nevertheless, since most of us grew up believing that we were descended from land apes, we can have an interesting shift in perspective to consider that we may be more like a dolphin, whale, or sea lion than an ape. After all, we share 99.9 percent of our genes with dolphins, more than the 98.8 percent we share with higher primates, including gorillas and chimpanzees.

You also have the more recent cellular memory of having been a fetus yourself, growing and moving within the amniotic ocean of your mother for nine months. Frequently, these memories are associated with great pleasure and security. What do you imagine it would be like to spend nine months in a water environment with all your needs met? Certainly, it would be an impactful experience that you would carry with you from that time forward.

Whatever the origins for a connection between water and humans, there does appear to be a high percentage of women attracted to water during pregnancy.[5] I have frequently heard women tell me that they would dream of the ocean and her sea creatures during their pregnancies, feeling the lightness and ability to move freely in the water that they did not experience in their waking consciousness and normal day-to-day routine, in gravity. One woman said, "It got to be where I was looking forward to going to sleep at night just so I could dream of being in the sea and moving freely with my baby inside of me."

Igor Charkovsky, infant swimming and water birth advocate in the Soviet Union, suggested that women consciously connect with the sea during their pregnancies, especially with images of dolphins or whales through meditation and visualization.[6] I journeyed to the Soviet Union and met with women who had practiced this type of visualization. They reported that they received messages through their visualizations from the dolphins regarding their pregnancies, even with specific advice about daily concerns.

Many women told me, and I myself experienced during my pregnancies, the pleasure of spending long periods of time in a warm bath, relaxing and allowing the water to support the weight of my body. This seems to be a particularly good time to bond with the baby in the womb and to give and receive those special communications between mothers and babies.

Water is also an excellent medium for fitness and cardiovascular exercise for pregnant women. Water and pregnancy seem to naturally go hand-in-hand for physical, emotional, mental, and spiritual wellbeing.

BECOMING PREGNANT

It can be illuminating for you to look at the context or process by which you became pregnant. To do so can make you aware of the richness of this magical experience, the creation of human life. To look at conception opens you to your philosophy of life—your relationship with bringing the unknown and invisible into physical form."Conceive" comes from the French word "to take in" and is defined as "to become pregnant (with young); To cause to begin: to originate; to take into one's mind; to form a conception of: imagine or image; to apprehend by reason or imagination: understand; to be of the opinion; to become pregnant." [7]

The Urge to Have A Baby: Where Does It Come From?

The desire to conceive a child can come from complex motivations, many times unconscious. To ask yourself the question,

"Why do I wish to conceive a child?" and to answer it honestly may show you some surprises about yourself or your partner. Once you examine your responses to the following questions, you will be better able to choose the context of pregnancy and parenthood that is most harmonious for you.

Where does the urge to birth and parent a child come from within you? Is it something you have unquestioningly decided to do because "everyone does it?" Is it the natural culmination of love shared between two people? Is it a way for you to be doing God's will? Is this urge to create new life from your own physical body simply a physiological, hormonal process for the preservation of our species? Do you desire to give to another what has been given to you by your parents? Do you desire to have a baby so that you will be sure to never be alone again? Or to assure your immortality through your children? Are you trying to please your parents or partner who want you to have a baby? Do you want to know that you have the power and courage to reproduce another being, that you can survive the childbirth process? Are you becoming pregnant because you feel a particular soul wanting to be born to you? Do you want a real, live little "doll" to baby and dress up? Do you want your image enhanced by having children that are a credit to you? Do you want children who can take over your business when you are gone? Do you have the feeling that you would not be a real woman or man if you did not produce a child?

The urge to conceive a child is undeniably present in most people at some time in their lives. What you do with that urge is a choice, no matter how unquestioningly preordained it seems for you to be a parent. To know that you are a whole, complete, fulfilled human being who has a choice about conception is a powerful position from which to begin to look at making or not making that choice, or to re-examine the choice you have made in order to bring it more fully into that which you desire.

There could, perhaps, be other ways for you to fulfill your urge to procreate and other ways for you to fulfill your urge to parent. The urge to create something is the same urge that produces great works of all kinds in art, music, writing, science, knowledge, etc. There is no end to the possibilities for that urge to create, to "birth" beauty, wonder, and value in our world. The conception, pregnancy, and childbirth process is a basic lesson in creativity. If you choose, you can easily expand your childbirth experiences into all aspects of creativity in your life.

In ancient, small-scale societies, children were more easily parented by all of the adults of the community. It was easier for an adult to "parent," whether they did or did not have their own children. In our complex and segmented society, children have become more like the possessions of their parents, and other adults who may wish to share in their upbringing may be viewed with suspicion. In strong extended family groups, children learn from grandparents, aunts, uncles, and older children. Today, the extended family gathers once, perhaps twice, a year, if at all. Because of the current high divorce rate of 50%, many children are parented by one parent or a stepparent.

Many people, both single and married, are choosing to adopt children, even when they could have children of their own. I have wondered if, at some level, the increase in infertility that many are experiencing is a way to see to it that the abundance of children that are in need of quality, loving parenting have more of a chance to receive it.

It is liberating to know that you have a choice in whether or not to conceive and parent children. To come from a position of self-love and feeling powerful as a human being in your own right allows the choice for childbirth to come from inner desire and knowing, and not because you need to do it to become complete. If you have not experienced this realization of self-love and completeness within yourself, I suggest you begin a process, either on your own or with a friend or therapist, for the purpose of integrating the reality of your own wholeness. When you have a strong experience of that wholeness within, you can use it as a source of strength and faith in situations where doubt and a lack of self-love prevail. Life is a moving dance, weaving fragments of yourself into greater and greater wholeness. In fact, the more you experience life as movement and change, the easier it will be for you to be a stable parent because stability comes from flexibility, not rigidity.

Becoming pregnant usually leads to becoming a parent. When you parent, you are parenting the growth and development of a full human being, not just the growth of their physical body. How do you feel about being a guide to your child to help them grow into a fulfilled and happy adult?

Conception

Whether a person is pregnant for the first time or the fifth time, the process of becoming pregnant (conception) sets the stage or lays a foundation for the type of pregnancy that person and their partner, if they have one, will experience. How, you may ask, does something that seems to happen so far beyond our awareness mean so much to the type of pregnancy a woman has? Most of the time, women aren't even aware they are pregnant until weeks after conception, and often, their partners are not aware until long after that. Don't the sperm and egg just happen rather accidentally to come together, even when couples have consciously been striving to conceive for a long time? Isn't becoming pregnant a rather automatic, mechanical procedure when it happens? Isn't it the same for everyone?

What about the stories of where babies come from? Do they come from out of nothing into something? Do their souls or spirits come from Heaven or some other dimension to Earth? Does a stork bring them? What did your mom, dad, or grand-mother tell you about the appearance of your younger brothers or sisters? How or why do babies with certain personalities come to parents with certain personalities? How come one baby is so different from another in the same family?

Conceiving a baby, in many ways, remains a mystery, in spite of all the light that has been shed through scientific inquiry on the actual physical process of conception. I encourage you to consider the questions above, whether already pregnant or considering becoming pregnant. The answers to these questions will reveal to you your own unique journey to becoming preg-nant, and will help you to see the stage you are setting with your beliefs and values for the taking in of a new baby into your womb.

Certainly, one can see that if the conception of a new baby is desired and wanted by the parents (not to mention the rest of the family), there is a high likelihood that the pregnancy will proceed more smoothly and with fewer complications than an undesired one. How many of us were accidents? Unplanned or unwanted? Or unplanned and then wanted? How many of us were not wanted until after we arrived? Or perhaps still do not feel that we are wanted by our families today?

Becoming pregnant can be accidental or can be the result of a process of desire on the part of the mother, father or other parent, and baby, which usually manifests through sexuality in the union of sperm and egg and the successful implantation of the fertilized egg in the uterus, or can be assisted by reproduc-tive technologies such as IVF. The process of uncovering and allowing desire for a baby to unfold and be fulfilled in actual conception can take years. Scientific inquiry has not yet taken much of a peek at the processes of preconception, which would involve relationships, foreplay and sexuality, and the quality and meaning all of that has to the real people involved. Becoming pregnant involves not only the physiology but the emotions, mind, and beliefs or philosophy of a person. Becoming pregnant is an interwoven process with many facets, one of which is physiology.

Actually connecting conscious desire for a baby with physical conception is a gap that the increase in infertile couples shows us is not as simple to close as it once was. What does it take for desire and conception to come together? What about the people who say they do not desire to become pregnant and yet become pregnant anyway?

Pre- and perinatal research shows us that many adults who recall their prenatal life, through hypnosis or other techniques, remember not wanting to come here and feeling forced or pushed to be here. So, it appears possible for babies (wherever they come from) to not consciously desire to be conceived and to be conceived anyway. Research with adults who have remembered their prenatal life has shown that many recall being wanted and desired by their parents and wanting to be here. Many have felt that they and their parents had chosen one another. Yet others have had the experience of not choosing to be conceived.

The fact that so many people become pregnant without the conscious awareness that they have chosen to be pregnant is an indication to me of the strong fear many of us have of our reproductive ability. We would rather have pregnancy happen to us as an "accident" than to face the creative power we have to bring forth new life and our ability to choose with awareness to conceive. This may be a way to not have to take responsibility for the beginning of things, but to kind of "jump on board" after everything is started. Once you're pregnant, you're pregnant. You either choose to accept or reject it and go on from there. Maybe this period of not knowing consciously that you are pregnant is a period of grace, which allows you to move through enough of your defense mechanisms to accept the pregnancy once you are aware of it. How many of you have heard your parents say, "We didn't plan on you, but you turned out to be a tremendous blessing to us?" Maybe this is a way you allow yourself to have the pregnancy you desire without having to confront the conscious part of your ego that sits up front and thinks it runs the show and says, "I don't want to conceive."

I believe that when pregnancy occurs, it is an indication of agreement on the part of the father (sperm), mother (egg), and fertilized egg (baby). The degree of awareness of that agreement can and does vary tremendously. However, if you desire to have the ability to actively create and respond to your life, it seems beneficial and empowering to acknowledge the agreement that does occur in becoming pregnant. Any other choice is to be at the effect of a universe in which you are not a creative participant. Psychiatrist Graham Farrant spoke about "cellular consciousness" as an awareness inherent in each cell that encodes messages about everything that has ever happened to us, thus giving us access to memories as far back as birth, prenatal life, conception, and preconception.

What is happening just prior to conception? Sperm, which are continuously being manufactured in the testes, await ejaculation, each fully packed with genetic material. There is a long journey of nearly eight inches to reach the place where the egg is waiting. "Not more than a hundred arrive in the neighborhood of the ovum."[8]

Each ovum matures in a sac known as a follicle. Unlike the

male, the female has all of the eggs she will ever have, right from birth. Once a month, an ovum matures, bursts through the follicle, and begins its journey down the oviduct where the sperm and egg may meet.

Films of actual conception show sperm swimming in organized rows, carried along by the special mucus secreted by the cervix only at ovulation. Whenever a sperm encounters something round, like a white blood cell, it penetrates it, seemingly showing the single-pointed intention for penetration that sperm have. In time, all but a few (3-6) have died off, leaving the remainder burrowing into the layers of the egg cell. The remarkable view that this filming has shown us is that the egg shoots out protoplasmic "arms"' around the sperm (possibly the one she desires) and pulls it in. This fact refutes the popular notion that the sperm itself actively penetrates the egg. In *Babies Remember Birth*, Dr. David Chamberlain reports, "Although the 200 million sperm that have been launched seem frantic to get there, the scanning electron microscope shows that once they touch the egg, they go into an extended "hug" until one of them is drawn in. The egg cell membrane then changes to seal out all other sperm. If this process is successful, as it is about 40% of the time, pregnancy begins."[9]

Shortly after the egg pulls it in, the sperm, which has already lost its tail, explodes, unfurling all the genetic material inside. There are 46 chromosomes, or 23 pairs, half from the mother and half from the father. If one of the 23 pairs doesn't match, the odd one is an XY pair instead of an XX. The XY pair produces a male and the XX, a female. There are thousands of genes in each chromosome, allowing for thousands of combinations, and thus, we each come out unique.

The first cell divisions occur at about 12-hour intervals, and then the cells get smaller and smaller. "During the first week of its existence, the new being floats freely in the secretions from the oviduct and uterus on its way down into the uterine cavity."[10] The embryonic vesicle, formed by the first cells, eventually penetrates the uterine lining "to implant the developing embryo under its surface."[11] Within ten days of conception, this tiny cluster of multiplying cells (called a blastocyst), barely visible to the naked eye, has made a slow journey to the womb. Here, the favored blastocyst—again, about 40% succeed—will find a secure lodging place in the lining of the womb."[12] The second week continues the process of burrowing into the blood vessels of the mother, establishing a spongy layer that eventually becomes the placenta that transmits oxygen and nourishment to the developing embryo. At this time, the baby is still a two-layered disc but will develop rapidly in the third week to have a rounded body, head, trunk, and umbilical cord.[13]

Setting a Foundation for Pregnancy

In what kind of context and setting did the "taking in" of another being occur? Was it a relationship of mutual sharing and joy? Was there domination and control, or force and manipulation, involved in the sexual experience? Was one partner desiring for pregnancy to occur and the other not? What was the age of the parents at the time of conception?

All of these questions can help you to discover the feelings, thoughts, and attitudes you have about conception. Perhaps your own conception experience was similar to the conception experience you had for your child. Conception relates to how you begin things, and often, those patterns tend to stay with you in how you begin things as an adult. By exploring your own conception and the conceptions of your children, you have the opportunity to bring into wholeness facets of yourself that you may not have looked at before. You claim your full potential by choosing to know that you were conscious, even at conception, and that your children are conscious at their conceptions. Whatever you have not forgiven yourself or others for concerning your own or your children's conceptions, you can bring into your heart for forgiveness now. Whatever changes you would like to make in your actual conception or the conceptions of your children, you can allow yourself to make through visualization and through communication, either silently or verbally with your partner, your baby in the womb, or whoever is involved.

THE FIRST TRIMESTER OF PREGNANCY

Webster's Dictionary defines "pregnant" as "Gestation; abounding in fancy, wit, or resourcefulness: inventive; rich in significance or implication; meaningful or profound; Containing unborn young within the body: 'gravid'; having possibilities of development or consequence; involving important issues; momentous ... full, teeming." "Gestation" is defined as "to bear, the carrying of young in the uterus; to conceive and gradually develop in the mind." "Gravid" comes from the French word for "heavy" and means pregnant. A "gravida" is defined as a pregnant woman.[14]

During the third week, the cavity that holds the embryo begins to expand in advance so that growth can occur. A "growth center" emerges at one edge, and a big rounded head and tail emerge.

During the fourth week, the body stalk joins with the yolk stalk to form an umbilical cord. An oval body appears with a body wall consisting of three layers: one becomes the sweat glands, nervous system, the spine, the muscles, skeletal bones, blood and lymph vessels, kidneys, genital glands, and connective tissue. The inner layer will develop into the digestive tract, the urinary system, and the lungs. Between the fourth and sixth weeks, the nervous system and spine begin to form, as well as the heart, face, and throat. The heart begins beating, and the circulatory system begins to function. At this time, the embryo is 1/8 of an inch in length.

During the fifth and sixth weeks, the developing eyes can be seen as well as arm and leg buds. "This is a period of 'design.' Arms and legs, body and face, take shape as though sculptured from the inside."[15] Cells are moving in currents that will give rise to the ribs. The embryo is now approximately 1/2 inch in size. "The first evidence that the preborn's nervous system is working is found in the activation of the heart muscle at five weeks and in measurable electrical activity in the brain at six weeks."[16]

The baby is growing rapidly, the heart pumping blood throughout the circulatory system. At eight weeks, the baby is over an inch and is now termed a fetus. "Everything is present that will be found in the full term baby."[17] By now, the mother has missed two periods. In the eleventh week, blood cells are formed by the liver and spleen, and gradually, this job is taken over by the bone marrow. The thymus and lymph nodes are beginning to function. During the first trimester, the sex glands of male and female look very much alike. After this time, differentiation into clitoris and labia for the female and penis and scrotum for the male occurs. At the end of the first trimester, fingers, toes, and nails are beginning to form, and the fetus is about two inches long.

The first trimester of pregnancy is a busy time for the fetus. Millions of cells are dividing and differentiating into physical matter that forms a human body, complete with everything it will ever need by age eight weeks. Your hormonal system changes rapidly from the system of a single individual to a system that is hosting the growth and development of another complete system within your own—gestation is occurring.

Frequently, pregnant women, even in these early weeks, have a special look about them. My grandmother used to call it "the glow." I have felt in these early weeks of pregnancy what I call a "fullness" within myself, and it is of a different quality than the fullness I feel when I am about to start my period. It feels more like a fullness that is not going to go away. This fullness may also be felt in the breasts, which may be slightly sore or tender. The woman's cervix also changes after conception and becomes slightly blue rather than its normal pink.

So much is happening physically, and yet at twelve weeks, the fetus is still only two inches in size. Often, women are critical of themselves in the first trimester because they feel tired, or emotional, or nauseous without any external signs of a reason to be feeling that way. Yet, at the microscopic level, their bodies are doing a massive amount of work, and their mental and emotional state is also in rapid transition.

I know from my own experience that women are not only hosting a new physiology gestating within them but also *someone* and his or her emotional, mental, and spiritual consciousness. You are definitely merging with an entire being right from the beginning. You have entered a commitment to literally be with someone night and day, not only in the same room, but also in the same body. Pregnancy is quite an extraordinary process in accepting togetherness. When we give up denial associated with pregnancy, particularly the denial that we have a conscious being within us, not just a body, we open ourselves to the opportunity for incredible transformations within ourselves—in commitment to relationship, knowledge of the power of our physical body, awareness of less visible ways of communicating, a sense of spirit and spiritual awakening, the ability to surrender to a process that seems beyond our control and yet is natural, and much more.

For some people, there is never a question about continuing a pregnancy once they discover they are pregnant. They either are delighted they are pregnant or would never consciously consider terminating a pregnancy for any reason. For many people, however, the first questions that come to mind in discovering they are pregnant are, "Do I really want to be pregnant?" or "Do I really want to have a baby?" Even when people have been desiring to have a child, they may go through a period of doubt and wondering. Once a decision is made to keep the baby, pregnancy becomes a *total* commitment, not just a partial one. It is not like a class you sign up for and then drop out when you don't feel like going any further. Pregnancy, birth, and parenting call forth a commitment from our entire self in regards to another. "Commitment" comes from the Latin word "to connect or entrust." As with other commitments, it is our choice whether this particular commitment brings us joy or a sense of restriction and loss of personal freedom.

In early pregnancy, at deep physiological and emotional levels, whether unconsciously or consciously, the mother, baby, and father are dealing with their relationship to commitment. A basic question is, do you have a commitment to life and to your own wellbeing? Enough so that you can not only take care of yourself but also take care of another? Considering having a child, or having one, allows you to see your commitment to yourself as well as to another. In choosing to have a child, you are saying, "I have the ability to respond to a child, to nurture and support this child into the fullness of becoming a human being."

Providing for a child's physical needs is mandatory. However, parenting is much more than that. You must also be conscious of emotional, mental, and spiritual growth and development, and the opportunities you have to contribute to your child's health in those areas as well.

In pregnancy, which brings up a myriad of emotions, you can experience much healing of your own childhood issues—you have the opportunity to heal the infant and child within you. I encourage parents to imagine what their parents went through in deciding to have them. What were their conception and early pregnancy like? Then I ask them to feel the hurts, incompletions, or gratitude that they become aware of and to forgive themselves and others as appropriate. I also ask parents to visualize for themselves what they would see now as an ideal or optimal conception and early pregnancy for them. *It is very difficult to give to your baby what you do not claim for yourself.* In claiming a loving, accepting conception and early pregnancy, you are able to give that experience to your child.

Common Discomforts of the First Trimester

Tiredness: Many women, even in the first days of pregnancy, become aware of being more tired than usual. Women usually attribute this feeling to possibly getting sick or to stress in their daily life. During the first trimester, the experience of being tired may vary from feeling slightly run down and needing to rest to the absolute need for ten hours of sleep per night. We need rest when there is a lot of inner activity going on, and certainly, in the first twelve weeks of pregnancy, this is true. Women who have jobs may find that they need to take short breaks to lie down or sleep for a few minutes. This is normal and supports an optimal development of the pregnancy. Women who have begun their pregnancy with good nutrition and regular exercise experience less discomfort from tiredness than women who begin their pregnancy from a fitness or nutritional disadvantage. Physicians, midwives, and nutritionists are able to recommend good diets for pregnancy, as well as diets to prepare for becoming pregnant.

In our utilitarian culture, many women are taught that they must see the fruits of their labor before they will give themselves the right to be tired and rest after working hard. This is not the case in early pregnancy. There is much work being done, but it is not visible to the eye. I encourage you to take good care of yourself with nutrition and exercise and to love and accept whatever degree of tiredness you experience. It will likely not last your entire pregnancy. In fact, many women report that they have more energy and stamina during their second trimester than prior to their pregnancy. Do not lose sight of the facts that pregnancy is about change and that the discomforts of early pregnancy will not last.

Nausea: Over 50% of pregnant women experience some degree of nausea in their first trimester of pregnancy. Some theories hold that this is due to a "sensitive nervous system" and some to a disturbance in the metabolism of glucose.[18] That is why the standard recommendation for nausea in pregnancy is to eat a light, sweet meal, or carbohydrates, right before going to bed and immediately upon arising. Some women never actually vomit but do feel nauseous throughout the day.

Once, I spent four days sailing and discovered that I felt much like I do in the beginning of a pregnancy, rather nauseous but not vomiting. I was able to function but had a queasy feeling that got stronger in cycles of three or four hours. We spent a good deal of time in fairly choppy waters. I was amazed at how similar the feeling was to early pregnancy. I began to make the analogy to myself as a little cell rocking around in the great big womb of the Mother Ocean with other little cells, all of us coming into some kind of arrangement or structure to birth ourselves from the ocean environment onto the land of our destination. I and the other little cells had to learn to move fast, to be in constant motion, and yet to have direction and purpose. During those four days, a sense of "moving stability" developed within me and my fellow "cells." By the final day, I was feeling little nausea, even though I was aware of being in constant motion.

I was wondering if the millions of little cells forming within the womb of the pregnant woman may have a similar experience during those first twelve weeks of pregnancy. If such an analogy is accurate, then the more the consciousness of the mother's body and the consciousness of the developing baby's body accept their movement and change within a growing liquid environment, the less discomforting the experience of nausea should be. It is possible that nausea during pregnancy has to do with the experience of rapid, sudden change involving an increase in movement within the body-mind complex of the mother. Sometimes food, particularly carbohydrates, helps to give us a sense of grounding during stressful, rapidly changing times. Throwing up would then occur when the sense of grounding or stability from eating is gone and the feeling of only being in constant motion returns.

Often, what you learn in pregnancy is that two seemingly opposing conditions can occur at the same time—for example, stability and movement. In fact, pregnancy, birth, and parenting are powerful processes of learning flexibility, openness, and acceptance of change. You learn that you don't need the degree of rigidity that you thought you needed prior to becoming pregnant and becoming a parent. Life gives you a lot more leeway for changes than you may have realized before becoming pregnant.

Another theory about nausea during pregnancy that I have considered is that nausea has to do with the acceptance of another's soul or spirit into your soul, spirit, and body. I feel that the "glow" that pregnant women seem to have has to do with having an increased amount of energy and light from the presence of the baby within the energy and light from yourself. For women, this involves a tremendous amount of closeness with another, and I feel that often, the first weeks of nausea have to do with resolving the need to be separate.

The first trimester of pregnancy allows you to go deep within yourself and perhaps to become aware of just how sensitive you are and can be. This is a tremendous "miracle" experience when you accept the changes and sensitivities that are occurring within you, or it can be a nightmare when you dwell on the resistance or fear of so much inner change. That is why acceptance of discomfort usually brings relief, and being rigid or stoic in the face of discomfort usually makes it feel more intense. We need the ability to persevere and continue forward in the face of discomforts, and we also need the ability to simply accept and feel the discomforts when they are there. Most of us have much more training from our upbringings in the realm of persevering and going forward than we do in relaxing and accepting. That is why, as a pregnant woman, your experience will tend to balance out the learning that you lacked in your mother's pregnancy with you, and of course, your later nurturing experiences as a newborn and child. Your pregnancy can help you resolve incomplete issues and feelings from your mother's pregnancy with you.

Possible Miscarriage

Two out of ten pregnant women experience some bleeding in early pregnancy, but only one out of those two will miscarry.[19] In 30%-40% of first-trimester spontaneous abortions (miscarriages), chromosomal anomalies are detected.[20] Ina May Gaskin also states other possible causes of miscarriage as including: "defective egg or sperm, unfavorable implantation site, failure of the cells forming the embryo to divide and differentiate properly, failure of the placenta to function, infections the mother may have, other diseases of the mother like high blood pressure, hyper- or hypothyroidism, vitamin deficiencies, malnutrition, diabetes, uterine defects such as scar tissue, and incompetent cervix (a cervix that will not stay closed usually after the first trimester)."[21]

Many women who have miscarried before worry about the possibility of miscarrying again, even though they may not bleed or experience cramping. Some women know that they have a family history of miscarriage and worry about this possibility occurring to them, even though they may have never miscarried before. I have heard some doctors talk about the new baby as a "parasite" that the mother's body must learn to accept. They attribute some early miscarriages to the rejection of the "parasite."[22] As I have stated before, most people go through some type of acceptance process, even if they have consciously been planning a pregnancy. Many midwives and mothers I have spoken with feel these early miscarriages are a part of a deeper wisdom that allows malformed fetuses or unwanted pregnancies to be released. That is why many midwives recommend acceptance of a threatened miscarriage when that is, indeed, what appears to be happening.

I believe that the parent's emotional state about the pregnancy and whether they want the pregnancy or not are important factors in the possibility of early miscarriage. Certainly, psychological and emotional acceptance of the pregnancy would lend itself to a healthy implantation and early pregnancy.

Occasionally, women miscarry even when they consciously want the pregnancy. One factor may be a low acceptance of their physical bodies as being *good enough* or *healthy enough* to carry a baby. Sometimes, women have been mistreated or abused either in utero, as a child, or as an adult. Victims of such experiences, understandably, have a difficult time accepting the health and innocence of their physical bodies. Being pregnant represents visible proof of themselves as sexual beings. Having their sexuality so publicly displayed may be more than they are prepared to accept at that time so that a miscarriage may result. *Every physical symptom carries an emotional, psychological, and/or spiritual facet.* (For example, a sore throat or a choking feeling may result from something important that you have left unsaid.) In minimizing the possibility of miscarriage, it is important to look at every angle. Often, working through deeper psychological issues and memories will allow the physical symptoms to disappear. Working to heal the physical symptoms can allow the deeper emotions behind it to come to our attention. Each facet works hand-in-hand with the others.

Commonly, when a woman has bleeding or cramping in early pregnancy, bed rest with feet raised is helpful. Additionally, analgesics or sedatives may be prescribed. If symptoms persist, a hospital stay with round-the-clock supervision may be necessary. Generally, it is considered that a fetus has a better chance of surviving premature birth after the twenty-eighth week of pregnancy, although younger babies have survived. In the case of an incompetent cervix, which must be diagnosed early on, stitches are used to close the cervix and are undone when labor is impending.

I have discovered that many women fear that they will lose the baby simply because the process feels so much out of their control. They worry that there is nothing they can do to keep the pregnancy once they have decided they desire it, so they hold on in their uterus, afraid to relax. Once they feel out of danger of the possibility of miscarriage, they do relax and trust that they will not miscarry. Often, this is when women appear to all of a sudden "really" be pregnant. Their bumps start showing, and they feel secure in their ability to keep the baby.

Use of Water during the First Trimester

For Physical Discomforts

The use of water in early pregnancy, or anytime, is entirely dependent on the intuition and feelings of the mother and what would be helpful and enjoyable to her. Many women have found cool or warm showers or baths to be invigorating when they are feeling especially tired. Some women take a cool (or warm, depending on the time of year) shower and lie down for a nap or a rest. Cool water causes the blood vessels to contract and warm to expand. Cool water can be helpful in waking up and feeling more present. Rest is important when you are tired, but activity can often be just as restful as lying down. Tune in with yourself when you are feeling tired and see which would feel most restful to you. Sometimes swimming a few laps in a pool can feel better than lying down.

With nausea, you might also find relief by floating or swimming in a pool. Sometimes, I imagine that the activity inside my womb is being matched by me being active in a larger body of water. I have actually felt less "seasick" by working with this image in the bathtub or pool. Frequent showers or baths during the day help give relief to nausea.

I would not necessarily recommend immersing yourself in a tub or pool if you are actually bleeding in early pregnancy. I would recommend consulting your physician or midwife for their recommendation. If you are not bleeding but are having some inner feelings of fear about losing the baby, I would recommend relaxing in warm water while listening to soothing music, and allowing yourself to see images of a healthy baby and placenta and a uterus that accepts the nurturing of this child.

Water is for your comfort and assistance in your pregnancy, and when you feel comfortable, your baby in your womb will feel comfortable. The baby already is surrounded by the fluids of the amniotic sac and may enjoy the sensation of you also being surrounded by fluids in your tub or pool. Being in the water myself always helped me feel more connected to my baby inside and allowed me to imagine what he or she may be doing or feeling in the ocean of my womb.

For Physical Exercise

In the past, many women used to be naturally more physically fit because they were working outside, planting, gardening, caring for animals, and surviving primarily off the land. In some ancient cultures, women would simply leave the fields when labor began and usually dig a hole in the earth and, with the assistance of other women, deliver their baby in a squatting position. Such women were more in tune with their physiological processes. Today, as a modern woman, you most likely have to make a conscious effort to stay physically fit. Sitting at desks, riding in cars, and punching buttons do not require the kind of physical exercise that keeps a body fit—hence the boom in fitness programs for just about everyone from children on up to senior citizens, as well as for pregnant women.

In the recent past and still today, there are myths that exercise isn't good for pregnant women because it may be dangerous to the unborn child. Jane Katz, author of *Swimming Through Your Pregnancy*, says: "This myth is based on the misconception that moderate movement or bending during a normal pregnancy will in some way harm the unborn child. This is completely inaccurate. The unborn child is well protected from injury by the abdominal wall and the strong uterine muscle ... as well as by the amniotic fluid and sac." [23] She goes on to state: "A proper exercise program has no adverse effects on a woman's reproductive organs. A woman's uterus is a very well protected organ, guarded by strong ligaments and surrounded by the pelvic bone."[24] Being a couch potato as a pregnant woman is just as unhealthy for you as being a couch potato as a non-pregnant woman. Elizabeth Noble, physical therapist and author of *Essential Exercises for the Childbearing Year,* tells us that women who stay physically fit during pregnancy are physically fit for laboring, delivery, and mothering the newborn. Furthermore, women who are physically fit tend to have shorter labors and easier deliveries than women who are not physically fit.

Be sure to consult with your physician or midwife about the exercise program you plan to use so that they can include it in the overall program for your pregnancy. If you are considered to be at risk in your pregnancy, do not start any exercise program unless your physician or midwife recommends one.

In *Swimming Through Your Pregnancy*, Jane Katz describes a swimming program for each trimester of your pregnancy and postpartum, and offers guidelines for family swimming. Swimming is an excellent exercise for most anyone, but particularly during pregnancy. She states:

> ... improving your ability to utilize oxygen during your pregnancy may directly benefit your unborn child by providing more oxygen for prenatal development. And swimming is the best fitness activity you can find! Swimming is a unique exercise because it simultaneously improves your cardio-aerobic fitness, strength, and flexibility, while avoiding stress and strain...You'll discover that swimming is a perfect exercise for you during and after your pregnancy. It involves a minimum of stress and no pounding or straining at all. Plus, the medium itself—water—is absolutely delightful! Its buoyancy will help support you and its soothing properties will relax you. Just think, you'll have that weightless feeling, which you will welcome as your body begins to expand."[25]

More and more frequently, there are water fitness programs, especially for pregnant women. Most water aerobics classes can be taken by pregnant women with some modifications suggested by the instructor. If you have your own pool, or access to one, following the programs in *Swimming Through Your Pregnancy* can result in an excellent and enjoyable fitness program for your entire nine months of pregnancy.

Especially during the first trimester of pregnancy, swimming and stretching in water are much easier than non-water exercise. For some pregnant women, it is hard to want to do much exercise, so working out in water may be a lot more appealing than on-land fitness programs. Exercise programs in the first trimester may also be much gentler and shorter in duration than usual. I always find that I feel much better when I do some amount of exercise in the first trimester, even though I may be feeling tired or nauseous, and I consider five minutes of exercise better than none at all. It is also wise to remember that you may not feel especially tired or nauseous during the first trimester, and that is completely normal also. I often used to feel that I wanted some signs to "know I was pregnant," and feeling slightly nauseous or tired would confirm for me that I really was pregnant. You can trust yourself, your body, and your baby to be pregnant in the perfect way for you. It is not necessary to have discomforts as a way to be sure you are pregnant.

If you have never exercised in water (and I include stretching and walking in water as well as swimming), you will be surprised at what a thorough workout you can have without feeling the stress and strain that you may be accustomed to having in out-of-water exercise. For several years, I conducted a pregnancy group that included water exercise, swimming, and water play activities. The women always left feeling lighthearted, invigorated, and good about themselves and their pregnancies. They were amazed at the ease and comfort they felt in the water and how much easier it seemed to be to tune in to what was going on inside the womb with their babies.

For Emotional and Mental Health

Water is a wonderful medium in which to feel emotions and have mental insights, thoughts, and visions. People who have spent a lot of time in water have discovered that they may go into the water feeling tension or conflict, yet by the time they are getting out, they are calmer, smiling, and feeling resolution of specific issues in their life. In my second pregnancy, I used to sit in a warm bath, sipping tea by candlelight, and have the most amazing experiences simply by relaxing my body and mind, and observing my thoughts and feelings. This process is often referred to as meditation. Time spent in solitude seems to be just as necessary to good health as time spent interacting and connecting with people. In our technological society, we often forget to give ourselves quality time in solitude. We may drive in solitude to offices etc., and I have had some people tell me they have had amazing experiences waiting in traffic. However, this is not the only kind of experience of solitude that we need.

Particularly during pregnancy, I find that women are drawn to quiet time alone with themselves and their baby. Allowing water to be a medium for this special time gives the mother the warmth and security of water hugging her all around and can be comforting, especially when so much is going on inside. I often find that I myself have feelings of being a child or baby when I am pregnant. It is an added gift that the process of pregnancy gives you the opportunity to review what your life may have been like when you were in your mother's womb. The stories, dreams, or visions that may come to you when you are pregnant are special symbols or messages that you can use to love yourself and who you are in more and more complete ways.

I worked with a woman who would spend her quiet time in early pregnancy crying in the warm water of the tub for up to thirty minutes at a time. At first, she did not know why she was crying—she cried because the tears just came. Then she began to feel awe at the task she was doing in being pregnant and bringing a child into the world. The process felt much bigger to her than she could imagine, gigantic and beyond anything she had imagined before. She often felt unworthy or incapable of this task. She would continue to allow herself to cry, and then she began to feel gratitude—gratitude that the universe was trusting her in the miracle of birthing a child. When she felt the gratitude, she felt like she was her mother, feeling the gratitude she had for being pregnant with her. Suddenly, she was aware of an infinite chain of women giving birth to children who became women giving birth to children. She felt honored to be part of this chain, and she realized that she was not alone in this powerful process but that many, many women had gone before her and that, somehow, all that they had done and learned before her would be there for her to draw upon. After this experience, which spread out over several weeks, she had no more nightly crying, no nausea, and much more enthusiasm and confidence in birthing the child she was carrying. As she stated:

> This was a remarkable and meaningful experience for me, which I don't think I would have had if I had not taken the time for my nightly warm bath and listening to myself and my baby. What a surprise to feel so connected and at one with all mothers! My tears seemed to be the tears of all women learning to trust themselves to become mothers.

THE SECOND TRIMESTER

The second trimester is considered by many to be a high point in the pregnancy for both mother and baby. All of the monumental initial changes for both baby and mother have taken place, the fetus has been accepted by the mother's body, the risk of miscarriage has passed (for most women), early pregnancy symptoms such as tiredness or nausea are gone, and the mother may be feeling a sense of self-worth and accomplishment in the task she has set out to do—that of bearing and giving birth to a human being. Many women feel a renewed zest for life and have a great amount of energy at this time, particularly feeling sensual and beautiful.

At four months, the baby is approximately 4"-8" in length with fully formed hands and fingers. In fact, it is at this time that thumb-sucking begins, as shown by intrauterine photography.[26] The baby's bones are also forming at this time, beginning in the middle and going outward to the end. By the end of the second trimester, the baby will be approximately 10"-14" in length.

Around 4-5 months, or 16-24 weeks, you will consciously feel the first definitive kicking of the baby, although the baby has been moving for quite some time. In *A Child Is Born*, regarding an intrauterine photograph, Dr. Sundberg states, "This baby looks as if it were treading water, which is just what it is doing. The amniotic sac is still rather roomy, and at every vigorous kick the baby turns round and round, floating now head, now heels down."[27] In *Babies Remember Birth*, Dr. David Chamberlain reports on the research of Sir William Liley of New Zealand: "Constantly shifting position to keep up with you, the preborn will avoid any sustained pressure from an instrument that the doctor puts on your abdomen and will pull away from anything pushing on a prominent part." Liley discovered how active and sensitive these little bodies are when he was trying to develop diagnostic and medical treatments for them in utero. "Virtually all movements of the mother caused a movement of the fetus."[28] Dr. Chamberlain, continuing to report on the work of Liley, tells us that there are sequences of movements the preborn makes. In talking about the rotation of the spine and legs, he states:

> This has been seen as early as the twenty-sixth week and is a feat that cannot be duplicated outside the womb for two or three weeks after full-term birth.

This demonstrates the unique advantages of the water environment of the womb that provides the unborn with months of relatively easy opportunities for activity and self-expression. In all such moves, superb coordination of the brain and body cannot be denied.[29]

If the mother so chooses, often during the fifth month of pregnancy, a medical practitioner will do an amniocentesis to detect genetic defects by withdrawing some fluid from the amniotic sac with a needle. Chamberlain reports the unusual response of the fetus to this procedure:

Prenates about sixteen weeks from conception were filmed after needle puncture by doctors in Denmark. Half of them showed a striking, somewhat ominous reaction: they didn't move for two minutes. Half of them also lost the variations normally found in a series of heartbeats. This flat, unvarying heartbeat pattern is also seen in very sick babies or babies who have been hit by a dose of Valium or some other drug ...What we seen here is not indifference, but a sensitive, perhaps shocked reaction to what has just happened in the sanctuary where they live.[30]

Prenatal research is helping us to see how highly intelligent our babies are, even in the womb. Because of these types of research findings, many parents are carefully considering the benefits and risks of various procedures used during pregnancy, such as amniocentesis.

It is usually a wonderful confirmation to the mother to begin feeling the baby's movements and to be able to tell a leg from an arm or the head from the bottom. The fact that a real human child is inside takes on more of a reality. My memories (discovered through regressive rebirthing experiences) of being a fetus inside my mother are that a whole new level of communication began to take place when my mother could feel my kicking, moving, and rolling. Women who are sensitive to the movements of their child usually become aware of certain types of movements in response to certain activities. I have certainly experienced my babies kicking a book or a plate off of my belly during pregnancy. My friend Robbie Davis-Floyd told me that her 4-year-old daughter Peyton loved to play poke with the baby in Robbie's "tummy." She would poke Robbie's tummy, and the baby would always poke her back (see Figures 1.1 and 1.2). But when Robbie herself would poke, she rarely got a response—clearly Peyton's little brother only wanted to play that game with his sister.

Babies have also been filmed holding the umbilical cord in utero. I have one vivid memory of playing with the umbilical cord. When I began to have the memory, I first related it to pictures I had seen of astronauts in outer space connected with cords to their spaceships. Then, I realized it was an umbilical cord, and I was inside my mother. I remember holding the cord and rolling around and around it and laughing. I felt such a pleasurable sensation. There was so much space to move in, and at the same time, I felt secure holding onto the umbilical cord. When Robbie questioned her daughter Peyton at age 2 about her experiences in the womb, Peyton replied without hesitation, "I laid my head on a pillow [the placenta], and I played with a snake [the umbilical cord]!" By age 4, she no longer remembered these experiences. You might want to ask your own child about their womb experiences; if you do, be sure to do it when they first become verbal, as over time, they may forget these experiences. Being with them in a bathtub is an ideal time to ask, as the bathwater may help them to recall their experiences of floating in the amniotic sac. Remember that any adult can recapture such experiences using the psychotherapeutic technique called "rebirthing" or "breath therapy."

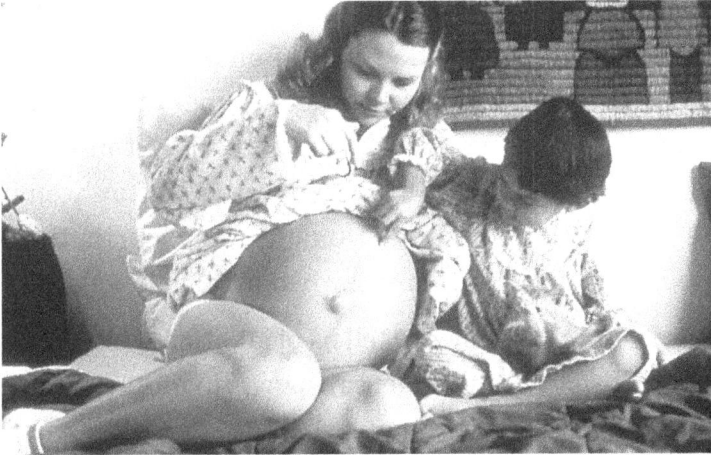

Figure 1.1. *Peyton playing "poke" with her brother.*
Photo by Peter Gonzalez, used with permission.

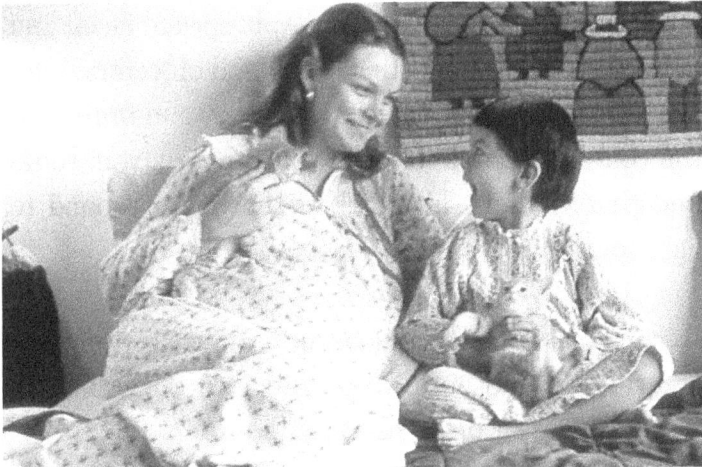

Figure 1.2. *Peyton's delight at being poked back.*
Photo by Peter Gonzalez, used with permission.

The prenatal experience had such an impact on researcher Dr. John Lily that he invented an isolation tank containing salt water in which adults floated, enclosed, for hours. People were able to experience deep peace and relaxation while being supported in this amniotic-like environment. Many people recalled prenatal memories and had visions of an inner world they had forgotten existed. Did you have an active inner world experience while you were floating inside your mother? Is it just as necessary for you as an adult to have supportive, secure womb-like spaces you can go into for rest and rejuvenation? Is that what you do when you go into your cozy bed for a night's sleep?

Chamberlain continues to tell us of additional pictures of the preborn that show an intelligent response to its environment:

> Squinting and sneering expressions have been filmed at fourteen weeks after conception ... Puckering of the lips, scowling, and muscle tension around the eyes have been associated with audible crying as early as the sixth month of pregnancy. Appropriate facial and vocal expressions imply that some kind of "central intelligence agency" is already linking body and brain ... If you could reach in and touch your unborn, you would find that virtually all parts of the body respond to light touch by seventeen weeks.[31]

In the second trimester, babies have been filmed actively breathing amniotic fluid in and out of their lungs through their lips. In fact, most pregnant women are startled when they first realize that their baby is having hiccups. Chamberlain states: "This liquid breathing guarantees that when the fluid is replaced with air at birth, the respiratory muscles will be well developed and capable of prolonged work without fatigue."[32] Research has shown that the mother's intake of alcohol and drugs slows the baby's breathing in utero, and caffeine and cigarettes speed it up. Both responses are considered to be efforts on the part of the baby to get enough oxygen. "These facts indicate that breathing is one of the first behaviors to be influenced by the mother's lifestyle and culture."[33] You do a great deal for your unborn child by giving them your own healthy, alcohol-, tobacco-, and drug-free body in which to grow.

Given a healthy, relatively stress-free environment for mother and baby, the second trimester is usually quite high energy with positive emotions. Both the mother and baby seem to be having quite happy experiences at this time. The father/partner usually feels the exhilaration at this time. No longer do they have a tired, nauseous partner but a healthy, vibrant one. Many women find they are interested in sex at this time. It is interesting to note that it is also during the second trimester when the baby's genitals are forming—up until this point, girl and boy genitals look much the same. Chamberlain tells of sonograms that have shown male babies with erections in the womb. He states: "What these erections prove is that the appropriate nerve pathways are definitely working by twenty-six weeks, something not previously considered. We can speculate that these erections involve sexual feelings and are prompted by something sexual. In all six cases, the baby was sucking his thumb during the erection."[34]

Certainly, sensitive parents who are willing to consider that their baby in the womb is conscious are aware that their sexual relationship includes a third person during the pregnancy. My memories of being in the womb during my parent's lovemaking are positive and natural. I remember feeling that the sexual experience was loving, fun energy, and I was lucky enough to be in the middle. Later, when I had my own room next to theirs as a baby, I wondered why when they had sex, I was no longer included. It felt confusing to me, since before, it seemed to be such a natural experience. Now, as an adult, I have experienced that same kind of playful naturalness about sexuality in my observations and experiences with dolphins, who seem to have a sense of innocence about sexuality that many humans have lost or never had.

There is an openness and acceptance about sexuality that you can impart to your preborn during this prenatal time.[35] Certainly, you are confronted with the opportunity to release any of your guilt about sexuality as you look at your sexual feelings during pregnancy. Your baby, who was (most likely) created out of the sexual act of union, is an organic and tangible part of your lovemaking. Communicating the innocence and playfulness of the sexual experience to the unborn can become a tremendously valuable part of that person's psychology.

The second trimester is an opportunity for you to bond with your baby in utero and with your partner. You are becoming a family unit as your pregnancy progresses. This is a good time to openly discuss your fears or concerns about the pregnancy or birth and the changes in lifestyle that having a baby brings. I feel that it is a particularly good time to share your feelings about sexuality. People often have programming from their own family backgrounds that either you are a sexual person, or you are a parent. The two can seem to strangely grow apart with the appearance of a child in the family. During your pregnancy is a good time to give yourselves permission to be sexual adults, as well as loving parents to your child. Maybe you heard from your parents or grandparents that it was wrong to have sex while pregnant and have guilt about having sex anyway. A good healthy, loving sexual relationship can only be a positive influence in your baby's life. It was likely your sexual energy that helped bring your baby to you in the first place. To all of a sudden begin to deny your sexual feelings just because the baby is present would be setting a precedent for separation between you and your partner, and at the least be confusing to your baby.

Another consciousness factor at this time is the thoughts and feelings you have about yourself as a pregnant woman or as one whose partner is a pregnant woman. What were you taught as a child about the beauty, acceptability, or unattractiveness of the pregnant body? Do you have some of those less positive self-images still lurking around? This is a good time to look at yourself in the mirror and keep looking until you are able to easily see your beauty as a pregnant mother. Most women discover that once they release old messages about the pregnant body, they feel voluptuous and beautiful, especially in the second trimester. During one of my pregnancies, I did belly dancing as my regular exercise program. It was astonishing! I couldn't believe how my image of myself as a pregnant woman altered as I felt the strength and grace of my pregnant body moving in rhythm with the music.

As a man, you may feel a great deal of attraction for your partner at this time. What an intriguing, mysterious process is unfolding right within her—a process that you helped initiate! If you can give up any cultural beliefs you still have about pregnancy being unattractive or that you may hurt the baby by having sex, you will probably also discover the tremendous joy and desirability in sensually loving your pregnant partner.

The second trimester is also a time when the pregnancy becomes obvious to others. It is a time when the fruits of your union are evident in your community. How do you feel about being seen as a pregnant person? Or a pregnant partner? Sometimes you may feel more vulnerable and in need of protection, but often you may feel open to being with others and proud of your reproductive powers. You may find that certain people seem to feel more uncomfortable around you and sometimes the opposite—they feel they can really talk to you or connect with you now. The fact of pregnancy will stimulate feelings and thoughts in others that you may be sensitive to, just as it stimulates feelings and thoughts within you that you might not have realized were there. This is another opportunity to accept yourself as a pregnant woman in the presence of your coworkers and friends.

Common Discomforts

Common physical discomforts during the second trimester are backaches, aching in the legs, or sometimes, constipation. The body is undergoing slow but continuous changes. The uterus is heavy, weighing on the intestines and causing strain on the back. Physical exercise is important to maintain and balance the body in its many changes. During my pregnancies, I experienced two or three days at a time that my body was stretching into a new shape, and I was able to support myself by asking for back rubs or lying down and stretching out my muscles. Constipation can be avoided by a healthy diet, particularly fruits and vegetables, and also by drinking aloe vera juice. Generally speaking, complaints during the second trimester are minimal compared to the first and last two months.

Uses of Water During the Second Trimester

For Physical Discomforts and Exercise

Use of warm water baths for back pain and body aches is beneficial, especially after receiving a massage. Water helps the tension to melt away. It is also a good medium for your partner to massage your aching muscles. He or she will have help from the buoyancy of water in holding you up, and you can relax more to enjoy your massage.

The second trimester is also a great time to enjoy and do your swimming exercise program. Doing aerobic swimming and breathing is a wonderful exercise for you and your baby. The baby will appreciate, as much as you, the boost of oxygen in its system. You will be able to stretch in water in ways that you cannot out of the water. This may be a good time to invite your partner to join you in your stretching and exercise program and see if you can invent stretches that feel good. You do not have to have an aching body when you are pregnant. Stretching, breathing, and swimming are excellent ways to ensure that tension will not build up. Being pregnant tunes you into your body. Your body gives you instant feedback about what feels good and what doesn't. Listen to your body. Your body knows how to move to release tension if you allow it. Continue to use Jane Katz's book *Swimming Through Your Pregnancy* and/or join a prenatal water fitness program.

For Emotional and Mental Health: Using Dolphin Imagery for Water Play

Our sea mammal relatives, the dolphins, have much to teach us about the ability to move effortlessly through life. I find that the second trimester of pregnancy is an optimal time for adults to pay some attention to these smiling creatures of the ocean. The dolphins can be a metaphor for what your baby may be doing in his or her swims in your womb and can help you get in touch with the pleasures of living in a water environment. When you have a "resident" who is living in a water environment within you, it is natural to want to know what it feels like to live within water yourself. Dolphins, who live in the water every day, yet are air breathers like you, can be great examples for you of how to play and have fun in a water environment with your baby, who is in your water environment.

You do not necessarily have to go to the ocean or an aquarium to be with dolphins to benefit from what dolphins can share with you. Simply opening up your thoughts and images of dolphins can allow you to do things in the water that you may not have thought of before. Reading books, seeing pictures, movies, or videos of dolphins are also enlightening. I especially recommend for pregnant couples the video "Commune with the Dolphins," which is a film of dolphins in slow motion set to music. It is about 20 minutes long, and there is no talking. It is a wonderful film to use in a meditative way that allows you to focus on the movement and grace of the dolphins without being distracted by words.

I also recommend using your dreamtime to consciously invite dolphin images and scenes to come to you. I did this after I interviewed enough women to discover that they frequently dream about being in the ocean when they are pregnant and able to swim freely, even though they are carrying a baby. There is a sense of freedom and grace that we are capable of experiencing in the water that is not as easy to access in gravity. Many women find that they are more aware of their dreams when they are pregnant. It is an optimal time to consciously work with your dreams. I suggest simply asking for you and your baby to swim with the dolphins during your dreams and see what happens. I also suggest that you ask for the most nurturing, loving support for you and your baby to come to you in your dreams. If you have specific issues or concerns, offer those up to your dreamtime as well. I think you will be surprised what simply opening up in this way can do to benefit you and your baby. Partners, of course, are welcome to join in. Dolphin dreaming can be fun for the whole family.

If you live near the ocean or have a way to actually observe or swim with dolphins in their natural habitat, I certainly recommend it. Seeing dolphins swim in the wild is a breath-giving sight and certainly gives one a sense of safety and comfort in the womb of the Mother Ocean—just the kind of image a pregnant woman can use when loving and accepting herself as a safe and comfortable ocean for her baby.

Once you have connected in whatever way with dolphin images, you are ready to enter a pool and have fun with yourself and your baby, and maybe a few friends will join. Then you have a "pod," which is what a grouping of dolphins is called. After doing some stretching, begin swimming across the pool, turning from front to back in a circle, alternating a front stroke with a backstroke. You may feel a little off-balance at first, but after a minute, your linear, up/down thinking will let go, and you will start to feel lighter and more open. Take deep breaths at this point and let go of tension. It seems that it takes a great deal of attention to maintain a focus on a linear reality—even though we are so accustomed to doing it, we forget that we are. Pregnancy, being a nonlinear experience, opens you to seeing yourself and the world from a more intuitive, less demanding perspective. After swimming in circles for a while, and if you are working with a partner, ask them to simply hold you while you float and breathe and relax, and just let yourself have whatever experience you are having. Sometimes, you may find that you will shudder or release fears, particularly of falling, while you are floating. Just continue to let go and allow your partner to hold you. That energy, or those thoughts of fear, are just what you need to release to open up to an even more enjoyable experience of your pregnancy and your baby. It can feel good to have your partner—or a friend—slowly move you around in the pool while you float. Try both stationary and moving floating and see which you like the best on that day. If you feel like it, you might try taking the time to share with your partner or hold them up while they float for a while.

Next, you can try doing circles head over heels, or the reverse, underwater, eventually allowing yourself to circle diagonally until you feel more like you are swirling through the water. When you swim, try moving both feet in synchrony as if you had a fluke, keeping your hands by your sides, and moving your heart and entire body in a wavelike motion. Experiment with the images you saw in your books or videos of the dolphins. Let go and play! If you are working with a partner, one of you can swim on your back, the other on their front. You can hold hands and circle or spin around one another, coming up and resting or floating whenever you desire. Taking breaks to simply float and tune into the baby is valuable. Women report that it is so much easier to connect with the baby and actually picture the movement of the baby when they have been moving and swimming in the water. You might receive telepathic communications from the baby. If so, just receive them and listen to your baby without necessarily having to figure out just how these communications take place. We humans, along with our dolphin friends, have incredibly intelligent brains. Being in water, I feel, allows us to tap into parts of our brain that we may have never used before. We have an incredible capacity to communicate beyond the face-to-face verbal communication we are accustomed to. Often during pregnancy, people can get in touch with this capacity to read minds rather than hear something word-for-word from someone they can see directly. Open yourself up to the many exciting and expansive possibilities for communication with your own inner self as well as with your baby.

THE THIRD TRIMESTER

The third trimester is a time of brain development and putting on pounds for the baby and for the mother, a time of creatively finding ways to be comfortable with the rapid changes within and to her body. Dr. Sundberg states:

> The last months seem very long. Everything is ready now; the baby has only to grow. From the seventh month until term, it increases in length from 13 to 20 inches and nearly triples its weight."[36] This is a time of getting ready for the "gateway" experience of birth, an ending of the pregnancy, and the beginning of life outside the womb. Dr. Chamberlain states, "In these last months, your body is pumping the baby full of antibodies, the disease-fighting proteins you have built up over many years. This is a gift that will go on giving, as a daughter eventually passes them on to the next generation ... In addition, the placenta produces gamma globulin for you as well as your baby, affording extra protection from diseases in the last trimester and after birth."[37]

At every level, both the mother and the baby are preparing for the exciting transition of birth.

The baby's heartbeats are usually easily audible now, often without even using a fetoscope, but by simply placing an ear to the belly and listening. It is exciting for the father, partner, or other siblings to hear the heartbeat. It is also easier to tell what position the baby is in, particularly after the baby "drops" and the head engages in the pelvis. Mothers and partners can usually tell where the baby's head, back, bottom, legs, and arms are, and frequently, the mom will get kicked in the same spot over and over again. Being on a steady exercise program usually helps the baby to go into the easiest position for delivery, head down, occiput forward. If a baby has been posterior or breech, or breech, they will often change their position right before birth. Floating face down in water and breathing through a snorkel is an excellent way to support a baby to turn.

This is also a time when mothers face their concerns about the size of their pelvis if they have not already. The hormonal system of pregnancy softens the cartilage and tissue of the pelvis, and women can actually feel their body opening for the delivery. You may have the experience of *knowing* that your body can birth your baby perfectly. You may feel that your baby is about to drop out, which is a good sign. Just visualize your baby slowly dropping out of the uterus through the cervix and vagina and into your arms. Imagine a safe and nurturing environment there to receive your baby.

In this last month, be sure you have a birthing environment and team that you feel safe and secure with. This is a key ingredient in readying yourself for birth. Often, there are last-minute communications you need to make, and there may be surprise changes in your birth plan that actually feel more harmonious to you now than earlier in your pregnancy. Trust yourself and your knowingness about the birth.

If you are feeling uncomfortable physically, spend even more time in the water, as you will most probably feel a whole lot more comfortable there, and/or get two or three massages a week. For heartburn, I suggest not mixing proteins and carbohydrates at the same meal. When I did this, I stopped having heartburn the entire last two months of my pregnancy. Eating smaller amounts more frequently is also a good idea.

You may also experience that you and the baby sleep or rest more often at this time, bringing all of your energy into yourself so you will have it to draw upon during the birth. The more you have exercised regularly in the previous months, the better you will feel in the last month. Just as in the first two months of pregnancy, you may not feel like doing much, but to swim or play in the water or dance and take walks on land can help you to feel as rested and invigorated as lying down.

Consciousness Factors During the Third Trimester

The two key psychological issues at this time are how you feel about and relate to making transitions, which can involve your relationship to transition at your own birth, and how much you trust other people to be with your baby in safe and nurturing ways.

In respect to the first issue, I suggest looking at your own birth by consciously finding out as much as you can about what happened. Then imagine how you might have felt experiencing the kind of birth you had. For most people born in the last sixty years, the experience of an easy, gentle transition was not present at their birth. Some common associations with transitioning at birth are pain, near-death feelings, being drugged, use of forceps or a vacuum extractor, harsh treatment by birth personnel, having the umbilical cord cut before you were ready to breathe, and separation from your mother. If you feel that any of these experiences were present at your birth, then you could re-vision your birth the way you would like it to be now, forgive your parents and caregivers for not knowing how to assist you in a gentler way, and affirm that transitioning is safe and nurturing for you and your baby. Hopefully, by this last month, you will have seen many films of many kinds of births. You might review the births you felt were the most sensitive and loving, and allow those images to connect deep within you and replace any negative images from your own birth or from the media, which often depict scary births in which things go wrong. Just trust that birth is generally a safe, normal, physiological and emotional process in which what you need most is an environment in which you feel entirely safe, along with skilled support.

Since most of us experienced harsh or unconscious treatment from the people at our births, we have a memory within us that says, "It's not safe to share my body or my baby with others." Many pregnant women go through a phase of not wanting the pregnancy to end but wanting to keep the baby inside where they know the baby will be safe and unharmed. There is a letting go of the pregnancy that occurs and a willingness to trust your baby out in the world. You can facilitate this process by visualizing birthing your baby with all the support and acknowledgment you desire. Visualizing a positive delivery scene will prepare your consciousness to allow for a loving, welcoming reception at the birth. Make sure your caregivers are on board with that plan.

In preparing for the birth of your baby, your physical body must be ready, and so must your emotional body. Gayle Petersen, author of *Birthing Normally,* states:

> A woman who prepares herself to grow during preg-
> nancy (both psychologically and physically) is able
> to make the most of the creative and transformative
> nature of pregnancy, birth, and motherhood. Current
> research has documented definite gains in self-confi-
> dence, and in psychological strength for women who
> have actively participated in the childbirth process.[38]

The totality of who you are is birthing the baby. In other
words, your mind must be open to the delivery, along with
your heart, your emotions, your spirit, and your physical body.
Particularly in our Western culture, which has emphasized
controlling the emotions, we are not accustomed to allowing
emotional energy to flow freely through us. We judge the energy
we feel and label it anger, grief, or fear, and then decide if it is
acceptable or unacceptable to express that particular feeling we
are having at that time.

From childhood on, most of us learned that our emotions
were unacceptable to express with other people. This training
in holding on to your expression of feelings will not serve you
in giving birth to your children. Birth is definitely not a time
to hold onto anything but a basic trust in the natural flow of
birth and your ability to allow this amazing process to occur
in a concrete way—through your physical body. Birth is also a
sexual experience. "Birth is an expression of your sexual nature,
and to give birth is to express oneself sexually. Pregnant women
need support in identifying themselves as sexual. Sexuality is
not an act, but a part of life."[39] Birth is not a time when you look

"all nice," all "put together," performing at your best. You will be beautiful and real and down to earth, but you won't exactly look like you're going out on an important job interview. I have seen many women approach birth like a performance in which they weren't going to miss a cue and would complete the performance in perfect order. That approach has not worked well, to my knowledge. It certainly is appropriate in some situations, but birth is not one of them. There is a choreography to birth, but it is open, flexible, and ever-surprising.

If you have difficulty in accepting the more "not put together" side of yourself, I suggest making peace with "her" through dialogue and visualization. If you can accept and love the part of you that knows how to be uninhibited and free without judging yourself, you will go a long way in opening a space for your birth to flow freely.

Make a list of the feelings and beliefs you have towards the "uninhibited, not put together" side of yourself. Then, visualize unconditionally embracing each one of the statements. For example, if you wrote, "She'd scare people with her wildness," let that statement come into your heart and say, "I love you thinking you scare people with your wildness," or "It's safe for you to express your wildness to me." If you wrote, "She'd be powerful," you could say, "I love and accept your power." Then as a third step, turn them into first-person "I" statements.

Use of Water During the Third Trimester

Water for Physical Discomforts and Exercise

Having a pool, hot tub, or large bathtub can be appreciated, especially during the last few months. By this time, you may be carrying 30-40 extra pounds of weight and feel that it's easier to roll around than walk. I used to spend time floating face down with my belly hanging through a big inner tube. It was the only way I could be face down at that point in my pregnancy, and it felt wonderful to just rest my head on the inner tube and let my belly go. Pregnant women tell me they are so grateful for water in the last months because it enables them to move so much more easily and find comfortable positions to relax. Many have also told me it's much easier to sleep on a waterbed while pregnant than a regular mattress.

Relaxing in warm water can help with backaches, leg aches, can facilitate easier breathing, helps to reduce high blood pressure, and is a way to have fun rather than being so intensely focused on "When is the baby going to come?"

Most pregnant women find that they enjoy continuing their water fitness and water play activities right up to the birth.

Water for Emotional and Mental Health

What I would be sure to include in these last two months are some therapeutic emotional release sessions with a qualified birth facilitator or breath therapist/rebirther, particularly someone who is experienced in working with breath and sound in water. I recommend sessions for yourself and your partner separately and then together.

When I work with a pregnant woman in an emotional release session, we include the baby in her womb and have an open dialogue with him or her. We basically communicate to the preborn baby what we are doing and why, and that the mom is letting go of negative experiences from the past to open her heart for the birth of the baby, and the feelings are not directed at the baby.

Surprisingly, many women feel they receive a response from the baby like, "Great, Mom, do it, go for it, that's fine with me!" When a mom is open to her process and releasing freely, I have always felt calmness with the baby. I and mothers I have worked with have felt the baby kick or give a more directed response when the mother is temporarily resisting the expression of her feelings. As a facilitator, I usually place one or both of my hands frequently on the womb to connect with the baby and listen to any responses, whether I receive them physically or intuitively. Often, the mother also places her hands on her belly.

It is important to work with facilitators who feel comfortable working with pregnant mothers and their babies in the womb. A facilitator must be clear of their own past experiences with pregnancy and birth so they can fully be present for your experience, not re-stimulated with overwhelming feelings from their own. So, don't jump in the water for an emotional release session with someone you do not feel totally confident about. It would be better to be with your partner or a trustworthy friend than to be with a professional facilitator whom you do not trust. I designed my Birth Facilitator curriculum to give therapists and birth professionals the safety and confidence they need to work with their clients on their emotional/psychological issues of pregnancy, birth, and parenting, in or out of water.

I suggest beginning your water release session with some regular swimming and breathing exercises, letting go of tension and worries, and opening to listening to the infant (that you were) within. I am imagining that you have a birth facilitator—who might be your partner, your doula, or a professional therapist—with you to help support you and guide you in this process, and that you have shared with them what you know or remember about your own birth. Perhaps you already have a focus and know that you want to examine the use of forceps or drugs at your birth, etc. I then would invite the infant that you were to be fully present in this session and to feel free to make any sound, movement, or breathe in any way that she wants. Give her permission to express anything that she wants to express with an agreement to not harm herself or anyone else. You may know immediately what wants to be expressed and how you want to express it, or you may simply want your facilitator to hold you while you relax and breathe and continue listening.

Generally, a water release session is divided into four parts: warming up by stretching and swimming for 5-10 minutes; releasing the negative or shadow voices within through sound and movement for 10-20 minutes; relaxing comfortably while quiet and breathing into the heart for 20 minutes; then revisioning the healed or whole picture in regards to whatever you are focusing on in the session. You may enjoy being held and floated or rocked for 10-20 minutes while revisioning. At the completion of a session in the water, I ask the mother or father to leave the pool and lie down on a mattress with towels or covers over them to integrate their experience for another 10-20 minutes.

Here are some examples of ways to release different emotions in the water. It is much easier and safer for a pregnant woman to release anger in water than on land. In water, you can move your arms and legs freely without endangering yourself. Often, simple little movements can facilitate a big release of anger. It is simply letting the infant through you, the adult, express whatever anger or hurt she feels. You may want to push at the water with your hands stretched open or closed in a fist. Sometimes it feels good to be able to kick out in the water or bicycle your legs to release energy. In no way would you be running into a hard surface causing a stressful impact to your body. All of these expressions can be done safely and with a minimum of effort in the water.

Many times with the emotion of grief, there is a heartbreaking scream that comes out of people, not unlike the sounds associated with a baby's cry (in a traditional hospital birth). You can cry underwater or scream freely without worrying about other people hearing and being concerned. There are times in emotional release work when you may want to cry or scream as loud as you want to without feeling inhibited. Water is a perfect medium for those expressions. Feeling comfortable and open in your throat area can help you feel comfortable and open in your cervix and vagina. Often, midwives will tell birthing women to relax, open their mouth, and make deep guttural sounds (or sing), and their cervix and vagina will relax also. That is because many midwives believe that there is an energetic connection between the throat and the cervix. Deep guttural sounds open the throat, causing the throat muscles to open, and thus, the cervix will open too.[40] High-pitched sounds with a closed throat can inhibit cervical opening. In a water release session, you may try experimenting with various sounds. Pay close attention to how you feel in different parts of your body when you make different sounds. Just take a big breath, put your head underwater, and let out whatever sound wants to come out. I guarantee that no matter how loud, piercing, deep, or resonating your sound is, people above the water will not be able to hear it. Come up for air again and continue the process. If you have recordings of the sounds of humpback whales, I suggest listening to those sounds before you get into the water and allowing them to stimulate your own creative expressions of sound. Try a wide range of tones from very low to very high and feel the vibrations in your body. Also, tune into the baby and see if you sense any communications from him or her as you are doing the sounding.

I often work with making sounds while I am swimming my regular laps. I simply let out a sound when I go underwater and come up for air and go back under, continuing my stroke. I affectionately call these sessions "swim and screams."

The third part of a facilitated session involves relaxing and being still while breathing and feeling the energy throughout your body, especially in the heart. During this phase, you may feel forgiveness towards yourself or others, where before, you had felt anger or resentment. When the negative is released, there is room for forgiveness and love. Your facilitator may give you statements of forgiveness pertaining to your issues. For example, if you had been angry at the doctor at your birth for using forceps on your head, your facilitator might say to you—or you might say to yourself, "I forgive the doctor for not knowing how to birth me safely and gently without the use of forceps. I release the pain I have stored in my body, and I set the doctor free." In this phase of the session, you may want to breathe through a snorkel, with a mask or nose clips on, so that you can relax face down. If that position is uncomfortable, try floating on your back with your facilitator steadying your position. You may ask to be stroked gently on your head, face, or heart area. Touch, in combination with warm water and your breath, can often facilitate even deeper letting go. In water, it's possible to be held, rocked, and soothed like a baby in ways that would be much more difficult on land.

In the fourth phase of your session, revisioning, you may wish to be held more in an upright position or with your ears out of the water. Your facilitator may rock you or hold you and talk to you like a newborn baby, making statements to you about seeing the perfection in the birth experience you had or seeing yourself born in the way you would desire now. In keeping with our example about forceps, she may say to you, "Your head slides out of your mother's birth canal easily; nothing is holding you back. The doctor knows you are coming out perfectly on your own and is simply there to gently lift you into your mother's arms." This is when you allow yourself to receive your heart's desires in regards to whatever issues or concerns you have had in your session.

When you are resting and integrating beside the tub, you may want to focus on the baby and relate the experiences you had to your baby. You may find that you and your facilitator wish to communicate verbally and share your experiences, and see how those experiences carry over to your feelings and visions for the upcoming birth. This may also be a good time to receive some gentle massage wherever you feel you need it, or to drink some juice or have a bite to eat. Take your time sitting up, standing, and moving. In fact, if you fall asleep at the end of the session, that may be the perfect way to complete the session by allowing your brain time to assimilate all you have learned and released. Just be sure you and your facilitator have agreed on the amount of time you both have for the session so she can wake you up when you need to get ready to go.

There is no one particular way in which people always feel after a water release session. You may feel relaxed and tired or relaxed and invigorated. Most likely, you will feel cleansed within yourself. I suggest being sure you do not have to do anything too strenuous, either mentally or physically, after a session, but plan to do something you enjoy that is restful for you. My experience shows me that using water to assist in emotional release during pregnancy is safe and gentle.

BENEFITS OF USING WATER IN PREGNANCY

- Excellent medium for stretching the muscles without strain.

- You can get a good aerobic workout with lots of breathing and circulation of oxygen to you and your baby, and move without unnecessary stress, as in jogging or walking on land.

- Excellent medium for water play during pregnancy with a partner, baby in utero, and other children already in the family. Often, it's easier to feel like playing in the water than on land.

- Comfortable, warm water is relaxing to tired muscles and a busy mind, and a good place to have quiet time for you and the baby.

- It is easy to feel connected with the baby in the waters of your womb when you are also in water. The correspondence of these environments is centering and grounding, and opens you up to easier imagining of the baby's experience.

- There is less weight for you to carry around. The effect of gravity is lessened by the buoyancy of water.

- Cool water can be invigorating, especially if you are in a warm climate during your last few months.

- Water is an excellent place to let go emotionally since it facilitates easy, safe movement, absorbs sound, and you can be held and floated while you breathe and relax.

- You can draw upon your connection to and images of dolphins, whales, and other sea creatures to bring ease, fluidity, and play into your experience of pregnancy.

RISKS OF USING WATER IN PREGNANCY

For women who are in good physical condition and desire to be in the water, there are no risks to appropriate water activities during pregnancy.

Personal Stories About Water, Pregnancy, and Birth

Personal Story 1:
Using Water for Emotional Release During Pregnancy

by Colleen Frayn, Mother, Chicago, Illinois

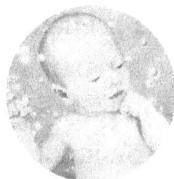

When I was pregnant with my third child, I decided I wanted to have a water birth. I knew water would feel good to me and my baby, but I myself was not comfortable with water. I felt like I couldn't put my head underwater without fear of drowning. From childhood on, I always had a sense of rigidity with water. I consciously asked Jennifer to help me work with my fear. She was confident in water and enjoyed water. We got into a hot tub on an outdoor deck. I lay face up in her arms. As I was breathing, I could feel the anxiety and terror within me. I was about four months pregnant. Jennifer continued floating me while I breathed and cried, and then gradually, I began to let her put me underwater. We were both working together, just as if I were an infant learning to feel safe in the water. There was no force. By the end of this hour-and-a-half session, I was able to go under the water without any help, open my eyes, swim all around the hot tub we were in, and come back up. For the first time, I began to feel real joy and pleasure in being in the water.

It may sound strange that I wanted a water birth and was afraid of water. However, I felt the water would support me with releasing the pain of labor. I had already experienced using a shower in my last labor, and it was great. I felt that if I could be totally immersed in water, I would feel even less pain and could deliver easier. I was unable to receive much touch during my last two labors, and I felt that being in the water would allow me to receive more touch from my husband and that I could lie in his arms and feel supported. I read *Magical Child* by Joseph Chilton Pearce, and learned that whenever you're going through any major life transition, it's easier to integrate when you have familiar elements around. Water and the mother are the two most familiar elements to the baby, so when the baby comes out, they are able to have those comfortable elements again to help them put it all together. I think right and left brain coordination would be enhanced in water rather than in an up/down environment. I knew in my heart that this was the kind of environment I wanted my child to have at his birth. I felt like the baby wanted a water birth also and wanted this kind of processing of my fear of water to happen. I knew I would be releasing the fear and would be helping the baby. I wanted to get the fear out of my system because I knew definitely that having it within me sub-consciously would not help for a smooth birth. I didn't want my fear of water to be a dominant factor at the birth.

Jennifer started out by pouring a handful of water over my face several times until I felt comfortable with that. Then we worked up to quickly dipping my face in the water. During all this, there were time periods of intense crying. Jennifer told me to just be with my feelings and was supportive. She suggested that I yell underwater, "I'm afraid of the water. I'm afraid I'll be suffocated," etc. I tried this, and the fear was less. After 45 minutes with her, I was able to hear my own inner guidance telling me what to do next. I would ask, in my own mind, "Where does this fear come from? What should I do now to help process this fear?" I would ask and get an immediate answer within my own mind, "Just open your eyes and swim across the pool."

Growing up, I rarely ventured into the water. As an adult, a friend was playing dunking games with me. Everyone else seemed to be having a good time, but I couldn't see it as a game at all. To me, I was about to be drowned, even though I consciously knew he wasn't trying to drown me. After that experience in the pool, my neck and spine hurt badly. Later, after I had my first baby, I got in a boat with my husband, friends, and child. I clung onto my baby for dear life. I was terrified the boat would flip over, and we would both drown. I knew these experiences were irrational, based on the meager contact I had had with water in my present life.

During my session, I had pictures of various experiences that I call "past life." When they occurred didn't matter to me. What did matter was that I was opening my heart to the pictures and feelings I was having and letting them move through me. I had a memory of being actually drowned, strangled by someone. I also had memories of my children being drowned. After bringing all these pictures and feelings to the surface and letting them come into my heart, I could see that those things no longer applied to this present situation. Previously, the terror had been immobilizing. After releasing the fear enough, I realized I could give up those scary pictures and beliefs. I used affirmations like, "I forgive myself for believing water is dangerous. Water can support me and my baby. I can enjoy the water and be playful and fluid in the water. The water will not drown me or my baby." At the end of this session, I could actually play peacefully and joyfully in water. I was even laughing and felt like a water baby myself.

Within the days after that session, I talked to the baby and asked him, again, if he wanted a water birth, and felt immediate movement in response. My own internal sense of communication with the baby was that he was happy that having a water birth was becoming more and more possible and enjoyable for me.

After this session, I went home to Chicago and was able to go swimming at least three or four days a week. I enjoyed exercising in the water as well as making up dolphin games with my children. I began to use a snorkel in my bathtub, usually lying on my side, to be able to be totally under the water and to focus on communicating with the baby.

When I was 24 weeks gestation, I started having contractions, pelvic floor pressure that felt like my bottom was dropping out. I asked my midwife to check and see if I was dilating at all, and she said my external os was a fingertip dilated, the cervix had moved to mid-plane, and I was 80% effaced, which should not be happening at 24 weeks. I was actually having preterm labor. Two days later, the contractions felt worse. She advised me to stay in bed and not pick up my other two kids. On a telephone conference call with other participants in Rima's birth facilitator school, I asked for support. There was a past lifetime memory that came up about the bubonic plague. I felt that I had been pregnant with the same child I was carrying now. In that memory, the baby was born early and died. The feelings in myself for the guilt I felt about my baby coming out early and dying were surfacing in my current pregnancy. I remembered that my whole family eventually died from the plague. In the release session I did after the phone call, I actually felt the dying and choking that was going on during the plague. I felt the baby was angry about that death and afraid he might die again.

When my release session was over, the contractions stopped, the pelvic floor pressure disappeared, and my cervix actually moved back into more of a pregnancy position. This was verified by the same midwife doing an exam a week later.

I took time every day to just be with the baby and talk to him, reassuring him that the past was over and it was safe for him to be full term. I continued to take it easy during the pregnancy but did not ever again have contractions and pelvic floor pressure. The midwife was quite receptive to my experience and the physiological effect it was having. The terror I had been having about losing the baby early left, and I was able to feel confident and enjoy the last months of pregnancy.

There was another way this pattern showed up in my present life. I was an RH-factor baby, and the third, who, if there is a problem, is usually retarded and can be born dead. The fear and terror from my parents, knowing this was a possibility, was what I lived with prenatally. I was third, and this was my third baby. I felt there was a correlation there.

I felt in using water to assist in my pregnancy, I was able to access clearer communications from my baby and my own intuition. Being in water seemed to facilitate that for me. I think it may have been because water somehow promoted me to be able to tap into being non-linear through the ability to move in all directions. I also feel that water is a great conductor of energy, although I do not know the scientific research on water as a conductor.[41]

When I would tune into the baby in water, I could actually hear Kent crying in the womb, and after I listened to his tears, I was able to hear words about what was going on with him and give him helpful affirmations.

Discovering how beneficial the use of water was in my pregnancy was a tremendous gift of the pregnancy for me. I now share my experiences with pregnant women in the hopes that they don't wait until after the birth to play with their baby in the water.

Personal Story 2:
Facilitating Colleen During Her Pregnancy

by Jennifer McPeek, Birth Facilitator,
Boulder, Colorado

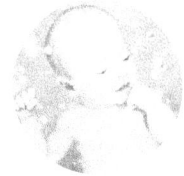

I worked with Colleen, who was 4-5 months pregnant. We did a session in the hot tub on the issue of helping her release her fear of water. I have always felt safe in the water. I began by floating her in the water, and that was scary for her to let go enough to trust me that she wouldn't have water splashing over her face and drown. That brought up a lot of fear for her, and so I worked more with her and started to rock her a little bit and get some more water splashed on her face. She would cry and release her fear. We did this process more and more until, eventually, I could dunk her head underwater. Pretty soon, I could roll her over and over in the hot tub. After about an hour, she was able to dunk her own head underwater and even swim underwater. She felt like this session helped her in preparing for the birth of her baby, and her whole creativity in general opened up.

An interesting synchronicity occurred during our session. Her son, who was one at the time, was upstairs taking a bath, unbeknownst to us. He was also crying and releasing in the bathtub with another facilitator. He ended up feeling more comfortable in water and being more playful. Colleen says both her sons were more comfortable and free in water after she released her fears.

I think for a pregnant mother to release her feelings, in or out of the water, is good for the baby in the womb. The baby picks up the mother's feelings, I believe, whether it's fear or grief or happiness. I tell the women I work with to sing to their babies and talk to them about their feelings and daily life. If the mother has fear about the birth for some reason, I think it would help the mother relax during her pregnancy and delivery if she would have the confidence to release these fears. I have re-experienced some of my mother's feelings when I was in the womb towards the doctor, for example, and know from my own experience that *babies are one with their mother's feelings*. I don't think it can harm the baby if the mother's feelings are released. I think the baby knows the difference between their mother expressing anger for the purpose of release rather than just being angry or in blame, especially if the mother will talk to the baby and tell the baby why the mother is angry, etc. and that she loves him or her. It teaches the baby, even at that age, that it's okay to express their feelings and that she loves them and they can love her even when she's expressing a negative emotion. I think that's important and just leads up to the belief and current research showing that babies are conscious beings in the womb. They really can participate, even though they can't talk to us in the language that we use.

Since I have begun to use water more in my work with pregnant women, I feel it is a safe and gentle way for pregnant women to work with their emotions. Water is so supportive and relaxing, and helps to melt away negative feelings. I also love the way water allows me to physically support the women, moving them and turning them in ways that would be impossible on land. I couldn't hold a woman and rock her while I walked across a room, yet in water, I can rock a woman and walk her across a pool. I think that type of experience of being held and rocked and moved is so rare for an adult and is beneficial. I think it rewires negative cellular memories from her own prenatal life or infancy.

Personal Story 3:
Dolphins, Pregnancy, and Birth

by Rima Star, Birth Facilitator, Austin, Texas

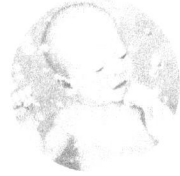

When I was pregnant with my first daughter in 1980, I would frequently have dreams of being in the ocean with dolphins. I would see myself swimming with them, pregnant like I was, but able to glide and move effortlessly through the water. In one dream, I saw myself as a pregnant dolphin swimming in joyous playfulness with several other dolphins, all who seemed to love me and the baby very much. This dream was so vivid that when I woke up, I found it hard to believe I was on land in my own bedroom in Texas. I did not tell many people about these dreams. I only knew that when I had these dreams, I would awaken feeling less restricted in my physical body, comforted, and connected with the baby inside.

I birthed that baby, my daughter Mela, into warm water and, during the next seven years, became vaguely aware that dolphins, being mammals like us, also birth their babies with the help of dolphin midwives in the ocean. I heard about "dolphin people"—people who basically worshiped dolphins and were eagerly researching their intelligence and behaviors.[42] My thought at the time was that I was on the frontier enough by talking about laboring and delivering in water; I didn't need to go even farther out by getting connected with whatever the "dolphin encounter" was all about. So, I continued to dismiss an active connection with dolphins even though I still continued to have clients relate to me their dreams of dolphins and sea creatures during their pregnancies.

One spring evening in 1987, I found myself giving a lecture on water birth in Sedona, Arizona. In attendance was Lydia MacCarthy, a beautiful blonde-haired and graceful woman (now I would describe her as dolphin-like). She came up to me after the lecture and told me she was an ethologist who had been studying dolphin behavior and communication since 1978. She said the dolphins had guided her to move from Florida to Sedona. I was amazed, since Sedona seemed to be as far away from an ocean as you could get. However, I did agree that it felt like being on the bottom of an ocean in Sedona. The water was gone, but the ocean floor was still there. Lydia said the unique electro-magnetic energies of Sedona resonated with the frequencies of the dolphins and their communications. She was there to open more to hearing their telepathic messages and to expressing them through her art. The fact that this intelligent and competent woman had so much respect for dolphins that she was willing to be "guided" by them impressed me. She talked about them like I might talk about some teacher that I admired very much. I certainly was getting the picture that these creatures were not your average "cute pet animal."

She said the dolphins had also guided her to meet me and find out about water birthing, and obviously to help me connect with dolphins. Lydia said, "The first week in June, I'm going back to Florida to see my dolphin friends."

Before I could get my mouth to shut, I had said, "Can I go with you?"

She said, "Of course, I'd love that!"

Part of my mind said, "Now you've done it, Rima, you're going over the edge." I decided, however, that I would go and not become flakey, as I imagined dolphin people to be (even though Lydia was certainly not a flake). Somehow, I would keep my earthbound wits about me.

In truth, I was excited about this new adventure. During the next two months, I thought of many reasons I couldn't go, but in my heart, I knew it was appropriate for me. At the time, I was facilitating a friend in her third pregnancy. Her baby was due in mid-July. When I told her about my plans to go to Florida and meet Lydia the first week of June, she wanted to go too. She didn't know if the research centers would allow her to swim with dolphins, but she wanted to go just to be near them. She wondered how the baby inside and the dolphins would respond to each other. Lydia thought it would be great for her to join us.

We flew to Florida on a Thursday, trying to be rather discreet while on the plane about Karen's rather large belly. Luckily, none of the airline personnel asked how pregnant she was. On arrival, Lydia picked us up, and we drove to Key Largo. She had arranged swims there at Dolphins Plus Research Center and also at Grassy Key Dolphin Research Center. We registered in our hotel, and by that afternoon found ourselves listening to the opening lecture at Dolphins Plus.

As I watched the dolphins swimming in their ocean pens, I felt awed by their size and their gracefulness. It still was a little hard to imagine that I was going to leap into the water with them. They told my pregnant friend that she could sit on the docks but could not get into the water with the dolphins. The trainer was telling us what not to do and what to do with the dolphins. As I understood it, the main thing he was saying not to do was be a bumbling, unconscious, grabby human being. What he was saying to do was to realize that we are guests in their living room and to be polite and allow the dolphins to come to us. He told us we were there as much for the dolphins' pleasure as they were for ours, and the more playful we were in the water, the more the dolphins would interact with us. The dolphins did not have to swim with us but could leave through a special opening into another area, off-limits to humans. He said that rarely happened.

We got fitted for masks, snorkels, and fins, and crossed over to the opposite side of the channel, where we were swimming with the four youngest dolphins. One had been swimming with humans for only six weeks. Each swim area was supervised by a trainer. As soon as we sat down on the dock, two dolphins came right over, heads out of the water, to put their faces near Karen's belly. They were clicking and whistling and seemed to be enjoying themselves very much. Lydia explained that their sonar allows them to receive an image of the baby in the womb, much as our sonograms do. Karen threw a ball out to them, and the games quickly began.

My experience in this first swim was astonishing to me. First, I found that I had quite a bit of fear when I entered the water. It seemed to be related primarily to their size versus mine. Dolphins weigh up to 500 or more pounds. I couldn't believe how small I felt with them all around me. Secondly, I did feel like a klutz in the water. It took me the first twenty minutes just to begin to feel like I could play. I was also frightened of them touching me. I thought, "They are so big. How could they possibly touch me gently?"

As I was more or less swimming through the water thinking these thoughts, I decided to try sending them a telepathic message just to see what would happen. My message was, "Please don't touch me. You're beautiful. You're gorgeous. You are so big. I'm scared. I want to look, but I'm too scared to be touched." I could hear them clicking and feel their sonar in the water. Every so often, one of them might come shooting by, belly up, a few feet underneath me. It was awesome. About one minute after I sent my message, a dolphin was swimming straight towards me. I thought we might crash head-on. Somehow I just kept swimming. Suddenly, about three feet in front of me, the dolphin stopped abruptly and "stood up" on her fluke. She proceeded to look at me, first with one eye and then the next, for what seemed to be an eternity. In fact, it was probably only a couple of minutes. I felt so much love coming from her that I noticed tears were flowing out of my eyes. The message I received from her was, "Don't worry. We won't hurt you. We just want to play." That triggered a distant memory in me, "Yes, I do know how to simply let go and play. I remember having such safety within me that I could play. Perhaps I could play once again!" From that point on, I was able to swim with my flippers in unison and even enter into some rudimentary beach ball play.

Karen and I both felt pleasantly zapped after that swim and were grateful to have Lydia as our dolphin guide. She listened to our experiences and was able to help us integrate them into a bigger picture of who we are in respect to this amazing encounter with dolphins.

The next day, we had swims at the Dolphin Research Center, where they did allow pregnant women to swim. Both Karen and I had an intention to ask the dolphins for any help they could give us in water birth and specifically in Karen's upcoming birth. We asked to swim with a mother dolphin, her baby, and the grand-mother dolphin who had been the midwife at that baby's birth. We were excited to have this experience, even though the time spent in the water was structured by the trainers into various activities. We felt that whatever connections we needed to make would be made, even though we would be going through various tricks with the dolphins.

One of the tricks they had us do with the dolphins was to go out into the center of the swim area, hold our hands palms down on the water, and wait for one or more dolphins to come by and give us a dorsal fin ride. This was tremendous fun! As the dolphin was pulling me back to the dock on one ride, I mentally thought, "Please take me around one more time," and she did. I was amazed! The dolphins loved clicking, whistling, and "com-municating" with the baby.

When I mentally asked, "What do I need to know to help Karen in her water birth?" the answer was, "Let us help you. We'll teach you about water. Water is a great place for human babies to be born!" I felt a sense of ease and play about birth that I had not experienced before.

Karen felt the message she received was, "Keep moving in labor. Let the energy of birth move you." We had heard that dolphins and whales spiral out their babies in birth, swim, and even leap during labor. We completed our day sitting by the side singing to them. They would slowly swim by and bring their heads up right beside us and listen. We felt content and knew that we had received a lot more than we consciously realized at the time.

We had several more swims with dolphins at both places, and by the time we were on the airplane taking off for Texas, I was surprised to find myself crying, with a flight attendant leaning over me asking what was the matter. I tearfully replied, "I can't believe I'm going back to Texas, where there are no dolphins swimming by my house!" I laughed at the words coming out of my mouth, and she laughed too. I said to my friend, "I've become one of them—those crazy, free-spirited dolphin people!"

Weeks later, Karen went into labor. She and I were both in her swimming pool, sipping juice with straws and swimming back and forth across the pool during the contractions. We were laughing because we were making these mooing kinds of sounds and had an image of swimming cows mooing in the water. It felt like we could just moo this baby out together. Every time either of us was in the water since our return from Florida, we felt like dolphins were with us, even though they were not physically present. It was a very comforting feeling, even though we didn't fully understand how this phenomenon had occurred.

As labor progressed, the primary midwife and birth team members arrived. Everyone was excited but also unified, since they had been meeting together for weeks prior to the birth. Karen left the swimming pool and went up one deck to the large fiberglass hot tub. Her husband was supporting her from behind, and she was in transition. Suddenly, a look of tremendous fear came across her face, and I felt her shoot out of her body, up into the sky. Then she looked at me like, "Wait a minute. I don't know if I can do this or not!"

I asked within me, "What can I do to help her?" and immediately saw an image of the dolphin midwife in Florida.

What she communicated to me was, "Go into the big pool and swim."

I said, "Karen, the dolphins are telling me to go into the big pool and swim. That's what I can do to help you the most."

She said, "Great, do whatever you can!" I left her with the other midwife and friends and walked down to the pool.

A part of me was thinking, "Boy, this sure isn't ethical—to leave a woman in labor and go jump in a swimming pool!" Nevertheless, I jumped into the pool and once again saw my smiling dolphin friend on my mental screen. What occurred next happened so fast that there were no words for it—it was all sound and movement and pictures. The image said, "Follow the whales." Her face disappeared, and an ocean of many whales appeared. One in particular was leading me to swim. I let go and began swimming through the pool in ways I never had and have difficulty describing. I felt like a whale moving through the water. Incredibly beautiful low sounds were coming out of my mouth underwater as I swam. I was getting lost in the movement and sound, and felt good. Suddenly, the message was, "That's enough." I got out of the pool, and it had been seven minutes. I went up to Karen, and she was much in her body and connected to her baby, whose head I could see beginning to come out. We looked at each other and smiled, and within three minutes, she delivered an eleven-pound boy with no problem. He certainly was a whale of a baby!

This was the first birth that I felt I consciously facilitated with the help of my dolphin experiences. I learned a deeper level of trust in the process of birth, specifically in water, and became aware of more and more creative ways to facilitate the opening of the birth gateway for our children.

Personal Story 4:
An Account from a Baby's
Perspective in the Womb

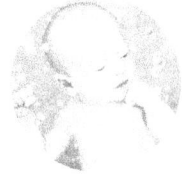

by Rima Star

For a while, I thought my mom was the entire universe. There seemed to be endless room for exploration. Then one day, I began to be aware of sounds that came from a farther distance away from me. When I became familiar with my mom's voice, I could then distinguish other voices. They did not vibrate as close to me as my mom's voice did. In fact, these sounds to me were music. I felt good when I heard them. I especially liked my dad's sounds. Sometimes, he would laugh a real deep laugh, and my mom would laugh in return, a higher laugh that I would also feel vibrating through me. I thought they were playing some kind of wonderful game, and I was in the middle.

It was fun to go places with my mother. For a while, I thought she was moving in a world of water like I was. I thought that's what the environment was for everyone. Then one day, she went to this place, and there were lots of mom voices, laughing and talking. One time, my mom stood real close to a lady, and I swear there was a thump on my roof, and I felt a voice say, "Hey, you in there. How are you doing?" I was amazed! Then I started to know that there were all these babies inside their mothers just like I was. Wow, was I excited! I wasn't the only one.

This one lady started talking, and my mom started doing things different with her body and with me. She must have been trying to reach the ceiling or something, and then all of a sudden, she must have reached over to touch her toes. Did I slide around then! I was lying on the rooftop of my house. The lady who was talking put on some music and I liked that. I began to rock back

71

and forth in my womb as Mom was moving my womb in circles. This was a new game for me. I wondered how the other babies inside their moms were liking this.

After a while, the lady who was talking said something, and everyone got up and walked somewhere different. My mom sat down, and the lady with the baby who talked to me sat next to her. We were so close that, again, I could hear him talk. He said, "Wait until you try this next thing. You will have fun!" What could it be, I wondered? All of a sudden, I heard this splishing and splashing as moms began to get into a pool. They were laughing and talking with one another. Then my mom jumped in, and that felt nice. All of a sudden, I felt lighter, like some extra force was holding me up. Mom began moving through the water, and I thought we were flying. Wow, my mom can fly! What kind of place could this be, I wondered, that can hold me up and my mom. We seemed to be floating above the ground, and I could move effortlessly all over my womb house. I laughed, and wondered if my mom could hear me.

After we did all kinds of moving in this big womb, someone came over to my mom and held her in her arms while she was floating on her back. I landed right on top of the placenta and rested my head. I was ready for a break. The lady was talking to my mom and asking her to imagine what I was doing inside of her. My mom said, "Well, I think she's lying down, resting. She's been working out too." I thought that was pretty good.

Then the lady said, "Is there anything you want to communicate to your baby at this time?"

My mom said, "Yes." Then she said right to me, " I want you to know that I love feeling your little kicks inside of me. It's fun to have you so close. I feel really lucky to be your mom, and your dad feels lucky to be your dad."

Then the lady said to me, "Is there anything you want to communicate to your mom at this time?" Wow, I was amazed. She was talking directly to me.

"Yes, yes," I said, "I want you to know *I love you. I love you with all my heart,* and I love having you listen to what I have to say. Let's do this some more!"

The lady said to my mom, "Did you hear her?"

My mom said, "Oh yes. I could hear her! She said she loves me and wants to do this some more."

It was good to know that my mom was just as happy with me as I was with her. From that day on, we began to have conversations, and they were some of the happiest times of the day for both of us. We went to our water classes three or four times a week. From that, I learned about play and being lighthearted, and feeling good about my body. I could also hear the other babies talking and their moms, and I felt excited about the world I would see when it was time to leave my womb home for the outside world.

Endnotes

1   Morgan, Elaine (1982). *The Aquatic Ape.* Briarcliff Manor, New York: Stein and Day, pp.18-21.

2   See Kanchwala, Hussain (2021). "Can We Communicate with Dolphins?" *Science ABC.* Found at: Talking to Dolphins: Can We Communicate With Dolphins? (scienceabc.com)

3   The only other primates that engage in face-to-face copulation are bonobos—a very friendly and socially cooperative species of chimpanzees, with whom we share 98.8% of our genes. As previously mentioned, we share 99.9% of our genes with dolphins.

4   Morgan, p.32; see also "Convergent Evolution" (2020). *Science Daily*. Found at Convergent evolution (sciencedaily.com)

5   See Balaskas, Janet (2004). *The Waterbirth Book: Everything You Need to Know from the World's Renowned Natural Childbirth Pioneer*. Thorsons.

6   Descibed in Ozhiganova, Anna, "The Birth of a New Human Being: The Utopian Project of the Late Soviet Waterbirth Movement and Its Inheritors." In *Birthing Techno-Sapiens: Human-Technology Co-Evolution and the Future of Reproduction*, edited by Robbie Davis-Floyd, pp. 193-207.

7   *Webster's Ninth New Collegiate Dictionary* (1983). Springfield, Massachusetts, Merriam-Webster, Inc., p.271

8   Nilson, Lennart, and Ingelman-Sundberg, Axel, *A Child Is Born*, New York: Dell Publishing, 1966, p.19.

9   Chamberlain, David, *Babies Remember Birth*, Los Angeles: Jeremy Tarcher, 1988, p.4.

10   Chamberlain, p. 40.

11   Chamberlain, p. 40.

12   Chamberlain, p. 4.

13   Chamberlain, p. 43.

14   *Webster's Ninth New Collegiate Dictionary*, "pregnant," p.927; "gestation," p.515; "gravid," p. 534.

15   Nilsson and Ingelman-Sundberg, p.59.

16   Chamberlain, p. 5.

17   Nilsson and Ingelman-Sundberg, p.79.

18   Myles, Margaret F., *Textbook for Midwives,* 9th edition, New York: Churchill-Livingston, 1981, p.153.

19   Gaskin, Ina May, *Spiritual Midwifery*, Summertown, Tennessee: The Book Publishing Co., 1978, p. 415.

20   Myles, p. 158.

21   Gaskin, p.415.

22   Nilsson and Ingelman-Sundberg, p. 122

23   Katz, Jane, *Swimming Through Your Pregnancy*, Garden City, New York: Doubleday and Co., 1983, p.5.

24   Katz, p.5.

25   Katz, pp.2-3.

26   Chamberlain, p.6 and Nilsson, p.92.

27   Nilsson, p.98.

28 Chamberlain, p.15.

29 Chamberlain, p.16.

30 Chamberlain, p.55.

31 Chamberlain, pp.5-6

32 Chamberlain, p.7.

33 Chamberlain, p.7.

34 Chamberlain, p.56.

35 See Odent, Michel (2014). *Water, Birth, and Sexuality: Our Primeval Connection to Water and Its Use in Birth and Therapy.* Sussex: Clairview Books.

36 Nilsson, p.143

37 Chamberlain, pp.7-8.

38 Petersen, Gayle, *Birthing Normally*, Berkeley: Mindbody Press, 1981, p.3.

39 Petersen, p. 49

40 For more information on the energetic connection between the throat and the cervix, see Melancon, Sarah (2021) "Safety, Co-Regulation, and Polyvagal Theory: The Autonomic Nervous System as the Missing Link in Childbirth Outcomes and Experiences," in *Birthing Techno-Sapiens: Human-Technology Co-Evolution and the Future of Human Reproduction*, edited by Robbie Davis-Floyd. Abingdon, Oxon: Routledge, pp. 208-221. See also Roncalli, Lucia (1997) "Standing by Process: A Midwife's Notes on Story-Telling, Passage and Intuition." In *Intuition: The Inside Story*, edited by Robbie Davis-Floyd and P. Sven Arvidson. New York: Routledge, pp. 177-200.

41 For some of that research, see Kara, Kelly and Suzanne Miller (2021) "Water as a Technology to Support Embodied Autonomous Birthing." In *Birthing Techno-Sapiens: Human-Technology Co-Evolution and the Future of Reproduction*, edited by Robbie Davis-Floyd, 179-192.

42 See "Meeting of I.B. Charkovsky with Esther Myers in Moscow." (1982) *AQUA* 2:14-18. Found at: Waterbirth | Birthintobeing; Sargunas A. 1985. "History and General Ideas of the "Babies- Dolphins" Program." (1985) *AQUA* 2:5-12. (In Russian); and Ozhiganova A. (2021) "The Birth of a New Human Being: The Utopian Project of the Late Soviet Waterbirth Movement and Its Inheritors." In *Birthing Techno-Sapiens: Human-Technology Co-Evolution and the Future of Reproduction*, edited by Robbie Davis-Floyd. Abingdon, Oxon: Routledge, pp. 179-182.

Chapter 2

WATER AND LABOR

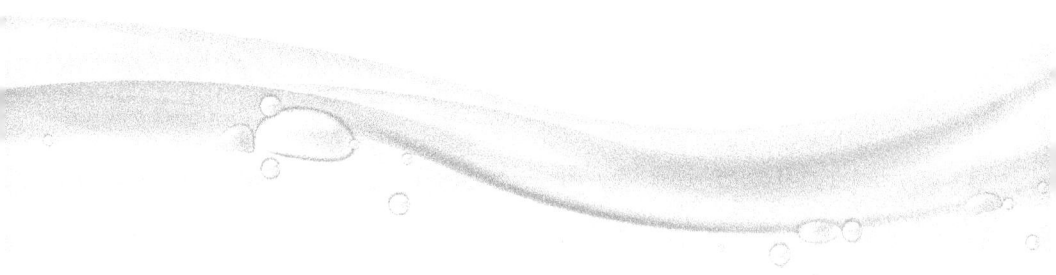

"Labor" is defined by Webster's Dictionary as "the activity of giving birth to offspring."[1] In *Spiritual Midwifery*, Ina May Gaskin defines labor as "the work the mother's body does after nine months of pregnancy to expel her passenger—the baby—and all parts of its life support systems (the placenta, its membranes and amniotic fluid) from her womb, down the birth canal and into the world outside."[2]

WATER AND LABOR

The physical activity of birthing is powerful work. The uterine muscle is contracting and releasing, much like in peristalsis, to push the baby's head against the cervix, eventually thinning and dilating the cervix to ten centimeters so the baby can enter the vaginal canal, where it makes a journey to the perineum and, pushing the perineum open, enters the outside world. This is a physiological process that, of course, is affected by the mind, the emotions, and the spirit.[3] However, once set in motion by hormonal triggering between baby and mother, it is an automatic physiological process that will reach its ultimate conclusion, the expelling of the fetus from the womb, unless impeded by resistance in the mind, emotions, spirit, or interventions from outside. In speaking about the delivery of the baby, Michel Odent states, "The fetus ejection reflex can happen only when the attendants are conscious that the process of parturition is an involuntary process and that one cannot help an involuntary process. The point is not to disturb it."[4] The process is somewhat akin to having a very large bowel movement or an orgasm. Once the triggering message is set in motion, the appropriate outcome naturally occurs. Midwives have long intuited what the authors of the latest edition of *Williams Obstetrics*—the pre-eminent obstetric textbook—have finally concluded: that the triggering message comes directly from the baby, who releases a signal to the mother's body that it is ready to be born "through blood-borne agents that act on the placenta or through secretion into the amnionic fluid."[5]

The predominance of physiology in the labor process means that women who feel the most comfortable with their body processes tend to have an easier time in labor and delivery than women who feel estranged from their bodily processes. As I mentioned in Chapter 1, women in some tribal societies may work up until labor begins, then go off to a quiet spot, perhaps with other women, to allow the normal process of labor to complete and deliver their baby in a squatting position or on their hands and knees. I am sure that if you asked one of these women to go into an institutional setting and lie on her back on a table to have her baby, she would look at you with shocked amazement. The fact that over 90% of all births in the United States are "unnatural," meaning that the normal process is physically intervened with in some way, testifies to the disconnection we have from our body processes.[6]

International speaker Michel Odent reminds his audiences that we humans are mammals, and that all mammals when they are in childbirth seek privacy. It is in this atmosphere of privacy with one or two experienced people nearby that Dr. Odent believes women are able to give birth as freely and naturally as possible (see Figure 2.1). He believes that mammals seek privacy so that the "uncontrollable activity of group members" will not interfere with the labor.[7]

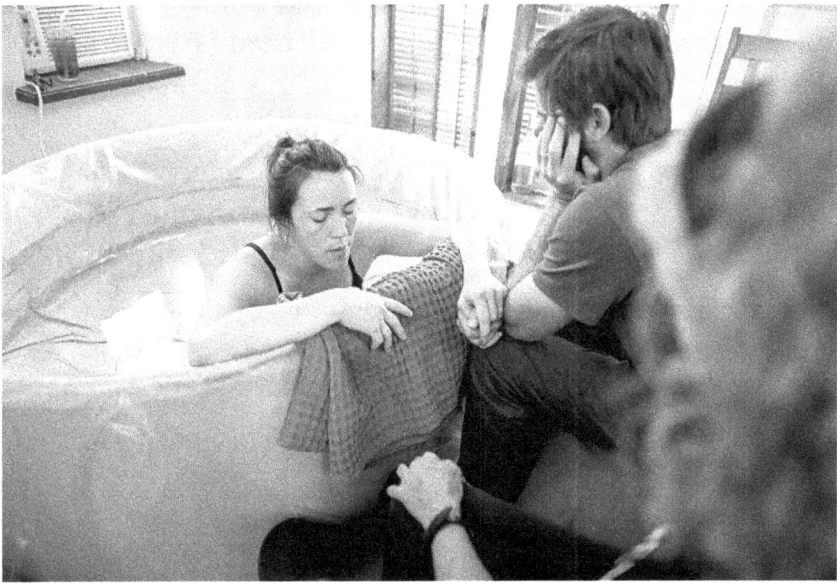

Figure 2.1. *My daughter Orien laboring in privacy with the support of two trusted people—her husband Andy and her midwife. Photo by Monet Nicole, used with permission.*

In our technological birth environments where interference is considered normal and part of being professionally competent, the need for privacy is barely noticed. Interventions can be of two types: those that generally impede the natural process of labor and delivery and those that generally assist the natural process of labor and delivery.

Interventions that usually relate to impeding or greatly speeding up the natural process of birth are connected with a mindset that views the body as basically antagonistic to the smooth delivery of the baby. These procedures include the use of drugs, like Pitocin, Demerol or epidural analgesia, the continual use of electronic fetal monitors throughout labor, and sometimes the use of episiotomies, forceps, or vacuum extractors at delivery. In a lecture, Dr. Odent reported that thus far, after numerous studies, the only significant finding in regards to the use of electronic fetal monitoring has been that its use increases the number of cesarean sections.[8] He calls this the "post-electronic age," a time when scientific evidence has shown us that an electronic environment has not been the best environment for safe births.[9]

Interventions that generally encourage or help the natural process of birth to occur are based on a mindset that recognizes the ability of the human female to birth without outside interference, and generally includes methods that return the woman to her needed sense of safety, privacy, and feeling uninhibited. Techniques like the use of dark, quiet spaces, the use of warm water in labor, gentle massage, warm herbal teas, soft music, walking with one's partner or friend etc. are examples of approaches that usually help to return a woman to her own inner world and knowingness about giving birth (see Figures 2.2 and 2.3).

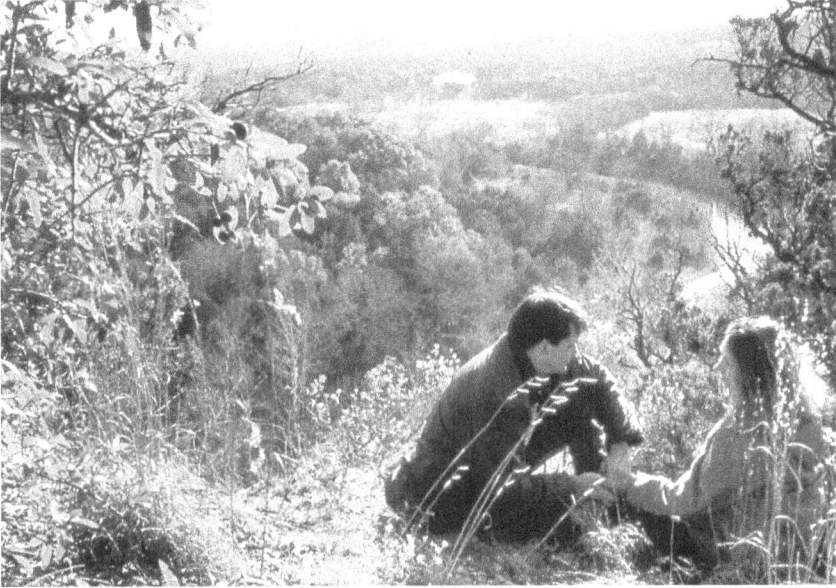

Figure 2.2. *A couple takes a nature walk during early labor. Photo by Peter Gonzales, used with permission.*

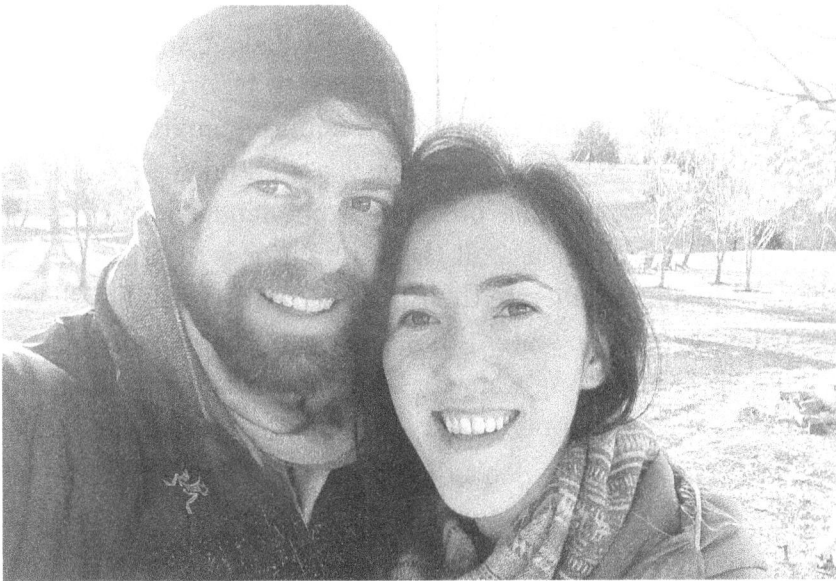

Figure 2.3. *My daughter Orien and her husband Andy on a nature walk in early labor.*

Often in modern society, because of the wide gap between an individual woman's willingness and readiness to do the work of labor and what her labor really needs to be like for the birth to occur, interventions are necessary. For example, a woman who is very frightened to open up her cervix and vagina could "fail to progress" in labor and end up with a cesarean section, which is a standard medical intervention for a woman who is not progressing, or progressing too slowly in her labor. In the United States, around 32% of births occur by cesarean. One of the primary medical indications for cesarean birth is "failure to progress." Yet active labor starts at six centimeters of cervical dilation; before that, the woman is only in what is called "latent labor," which can safely take many hours or days. Hospitals usually do not recognize the difference between latent and active labor, and so often admit laboring women and put them on a clock far too soon. Thus millions of cesareans are performed every year for "failure to progress" on women who are not even yet in real labor![10] In addition, Dr. Odent states: "There are few hospitals where the importance to laboring women of privacy, darkness, and silence, of a feminine environment, of the freedom to move and to be noisy, are all taken into consideration. But even in those hospitals, some modern women still find it difficult to release all their inhibitions. In other words, they are unable to liberate their instincts. Water can be a help." Dr. Odent goes on to state, "I have no doubt that a contribution can be made [by using water in labor] towards controlling the epidemic of caesareans that has insidiously invaded the industrialized world."[11]

The integration of psychological, emotional and physiological preparation prior to labor can help a woman trust her body and the natural process of labor and delivery. Believing and knowing, in a very physical sense, that you can labor and deliver naturally is very important to actually having that experience. Gayle Petersen states:

> A woman who has developed a style during her life-time of being able to meet and handle stress, without creating distress for herself, will be less likely to create blocks for herself in labor. Acceptance is the first step forward in the labor process. Acceptance of pain, of the work presented by the foreseen task of actively giving birth, of journeying with the baby towards birth, smooths the way for a progressive, natural labor.

Peterson goes on to say, *"as a woman lives, so shall she give birth."* [12]

In many ways it is a shame that we even need to ask the question, "Can I deliver naturally?" for it shows us how we have not kept our technological advances in balance with the ancient, evolutionary wisdom of our natural processes.[13] Another fact that indicates the wide discrepancy between natural birth and technological birth is the alarmingly high cesarean rate in the United States of 32%. The rate that the World Health Organization says countries should strive for is around 10%-15%.[14] Below that rate, women die from lack of access to cesareans; above that rate, women and babies suffer from the overuse of cesareans. The aim of this book and many others is to remind you of the wisdom of the natural process of labor and delivery, while at the same time not throwing out the gains of technological knowledge. Technology should be at the service of the natural process of birth and not the other way around (see Figure 2.4).

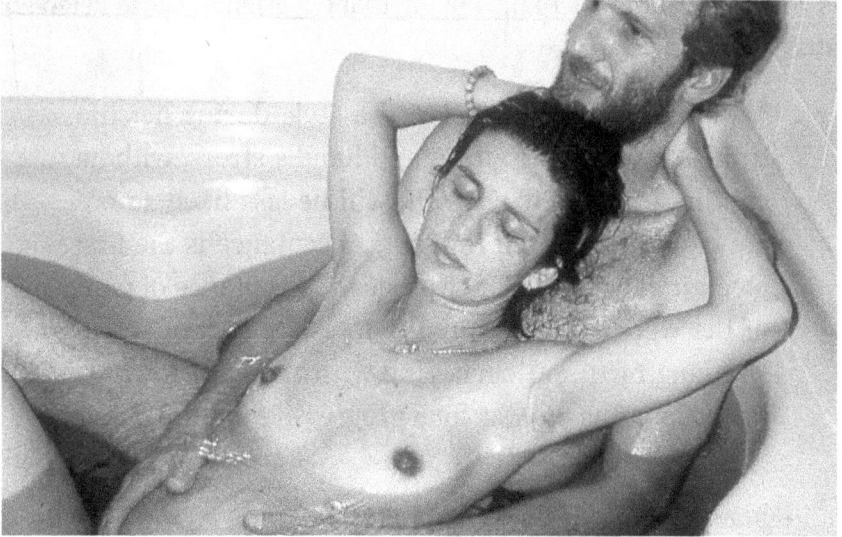

Figure 2.4. *Technology at the service of the birthing couple. But where is the technology? It is, of course, this highly sophisticated jacuzzi, the maze of pipes that bring the water, and the electricity that warms that water. Technologies that are truly supportive of birth tend to recede into the background and go unnoticed, while the laboring woman is in the foreground. Photo taken in Brazil by obstetrician Adailton Salvatore, used with permission.*

The use of water in labor is an intervention that generally assists the natural flow of the birth process. For many women, it is also the medium in which they feel the most supported to deliver their baby. Water offers a natural form of pain relief for laboring women, and water labor is more widely accepted in hospitals and by physicians than is water delivery at this time. However, hospitals and birth centers that begin to use tubs for labor should be prepared for the possibility of water delivery. Quite often there is no time to move the mother before the delivery of the baby, and frequently women will want to remain where they are.

Professional midwives frequently recommend the use of warm water during labor. When I gave birth in a hospital in 1968, I was given injections of a pain relief medication. At the time, I swore it did nothing, and once yelled at the nurse that the injections did nothing for the pain. In 1980, while birthing my daughter at home, I got into a tub of warm water when I felt pain very intensely. I was amazed at how much relief I felt. There was no comparison between that experience of pain relief and my previous one in the hospital with drugs. Since that time, I have spoken with many women who have had a previous medicated labor and then labored in water, and they share the same feeling. The relief they experienced from laboring in warm water was significantly more than the relief they experienced from drugs, with the exception of epidurals. Although epidurals do usually provide total relief from pain, they bring with them their own set of problems. These include slowing down labor if given before six centimeters—again, the beginning of active labor—and inhibiting movement, which is the essence of a healthy physiologic labor.[15]

Water not only helps in relieving pain in labor but also provides a great medium for a woman to be active in labor and move in many ways. Providing the tub is large enough, a woman can roll, stretch, float, and move her body into comfortable positions, many of which are impossible on land. Water also helps the partner or doula to assist the mother by making it easier to hold her or to float her in various positions. In my vision of a birthing center, I see a special pool for laboring women that is large enough for several laboring women at a time and their partners. I think sharing the experience of labor with other laboring women may be a helpful option at a certain point in labor, particularly with women who are looking for outside validation for their experience. Instead of getting this validation from authorities, let them get it from other laboring women themselves. I would certainly have smaller individual tubs available as well.

So much of the "work" of labor is the ability to relax all the parts of the body that don't need to be in use during the ebb and flow of contractions. Contractions happen automatically, unless they are Pitocin-induced. To allow the rest of the body to relax in the presence of the uterus, cervix, and pelvic floor doing their work is no small matter, but it allows the body to function in its own natural rhythm without resistance from the rest of the body. Water, which for most people is a symbol for relaxation, can be very helpful in reminding a woman to let go into the work her body is doing, to flow with labor and not to resist it. "What you resist, persists" is a popular saying among psychotherapists. Michel Odent postulates, "It is also possible that warm water acts directly on the muscular system. Tendons are composed mainly of collagen, and the warmer the temperature, the softer the collagen becomes. So a warm bath might have a direct relaxing effect."[16] Listening to the sound of running water either in actuality or on a recording can also be very soothing. In fact, Michel Odent reports that women in the hospital at Pithiviers, France, where he began his journey into water labor and birth, would progress very rapidly in labor just listening to the sound of the running water filling the tub.

Dr. Michael J. Rosenthal, founder of the Family Birthing Center in Upland, California, states:

> The use of warm water for labor and birth might be viewed as radical and new in the human experience. However, from a long historical perspective, the use of most obstetric interventions such as spinal or epidural anesthesia, narcotics, and forceps, are also very recent. No other intervention can be said to be so free

of risk. If the bath had been used earlier in this century, we might never have passed through the era of "twilight sleep" sedation that often depressed babies and removed women from conscious participation in birth.[17]

Dr. Michel Odent states, "There are no simple formulas for the use of water during labour. It is not a method that can be evaluated by 'double-blind' studies. The attraction to water during labour varies considerably from one woman to another. It can be neither measured nor forecast. There is no parallel with an attraction to water in daily life."[18]

Water is a very simple, relatively inexpensive alternative to more costly and complicated interventions for a painful labor, and it also affords a woman comfort and ease of movement during labor. For women who do not experience labor as particularly painful, water offers a pleasurable and soothing medium for themselves and their partners to enjoy.

IMPENDING LABOR

The whole of pregnancy is the activity of labor; however, the signs for the coming birth increase as the end of the pregnancy draws near. Frequently, particularly in first births, "lightening" occurs. Lightening is the baby dropping down into position in the pelvis so there is actually more room in the mother's upper rib cage and more pressure from the baby's head on the pelvic floor. Periodic contractions (which occur normally all during pregnancy) increase in intensity, with more awareness that they are actually "doing something" to thin and open the cervix. Women may lose their mucous plug many days before actual active labor begins. This plug has sealed the cervix during the last nine months. If the mucous is slightly pink or red, this indicates that the tiny capillaries of the cervix have begun to burst with the dilation and effacement.

Sometimes in the last week or two, a woman may experience what is termed "false" labor. These contractions are definitely not false—they are very real and important. A better term might be "warm-up" or "preparatory" contractions—also known as Braxton-Hicks contractions. The difference between these contractions and those of early labor is simply that these eventually come to a stop. With these warm-up contractions, you may want to sit in a warm bath and breathe and relax with them, and allow yourself to give in to a deeper level of surrender to the process of labor. After all, when they occur, you don't know for sure if they are warmups or if they will build into active labor. This is a good time to let yourself imagine how you would feel going into stronger, more intense, and more continuous contractions. Pre-labor contractions are usually 10 to 20 minutes apart and irregular, while true labor contractions are initially 5-7 minutes apart and quite regular. However, all of them are contractions that strengthen the uterine muscles and help to dilate and open the cervix for the passage of the baby into the birth canal. When I was having three to four hours of pre-labor contractions with my daughter Mela, I found it a good time to share my fears with my partner. It was a good completion in facing my fear that I would fail, wouldn't be up to the task, or wouldn't be able to let go into the pain. Sharing these fears verbally helped me to be ready for the beginning of actual labor when it occurred a week later.

Another sign of impending labor is the leaking of amniotic fluid or a gushing of a lot of fluid from the breaking of the amniotic sac. If this occurs, it could still be a day or two before active labor starts; however, it usually starts within 24 hours. With the rupture of the bag of waters, you must remember that there is now a channel into the sac that previously was not there. Obstetricians point out that the risk of infection is greater after the waters break, although many approve of standing in a warm shower. However, in the thousands of water labors and deliveries that have occurred in many countries, there has been nothing to prove that risk of infection is any greater than prior to the waters breaking. Michel Odent comments on this concern:

> It is strange that doctors who do not hesitate to rupture membranes, to repeatedly carry out vaginal examinations and to insert catheters or electrodes are frightened by the idea that a labouring woman might have a bath... it is obvious that fear of infection is not inspired by the facts...When the mother-to-be enters the bath at the stage of hard labour, she is not likely to stay in the water long enough to make the reproduction of germs possible. Also, the vagina is much more waterproof than is commonly thought. Dangerous germs are not in tap water. And finally, the use of water avoids some obstetric interventions such as forceps, vacuum extraction and Caesarean, which bring their own risk of infection.[19]

I myself have sat in warm water with amniotic fluids leaking, have certainly been in water when the amniotic sac burst, and have had no infections. I felt that the water was no more dangerous than the risk of infection from germs in the air. Many women find that using water during the time of impending labor is very beneficial. However, as always, it is up to the discretion of the mother.

FIRST STAGE OF LABOR

The "first stage" of labor is defined as everything from the first contractions until 10 centimeters dilation, when the cervix is open enough for the baby's head to go through. The "second stage" of labor is defined as starting with pushing. Included in the first stage is early or "latent" labor, 0-6 centimeters, active labor, 6-8 centimeters, and transition, 8-10 centimeters. Of course, these designations are arbitrary and simply a helpful model for birth professionals. Along with the increase in cervical opening are shifts in hormonal levels, emotions, and attitudes. Generally, the time span for latent labor is around 6-12 hours for a first birth, though, again, it can last much longer—even several days—and considerably less for subsequent births. Doctors usually do not recognize the fact that latent labor may last anywhere from 30 minutes to days. So, as I mentioned above, if you go to the hospital in latent labor, you may very well receive labor augmentation with Pitocin and end up with a cesarean section for "failure to progess," as in hospitals, the clock starts ticking the moment you walk in the door. But if you wait till active labor (again, defined as beginning at 6 cm dilation), you are much more likely to have a normal, vaginal birth. It is important to know what your doctor, midwife, hospital, or birth center's standards are. I have known some women who have a long early labor phase of two days or more in which contractions are definitely present before they actually click into active labor.

Immersion in warm water can assist a smooth transition through all the phases of early labor. Many women have chosen to use water throughout their entire labor, some sporadically and some at key points of intensity. There is not necessarily one recommended method for using water to assist in the first stage of labor. However, if contractions are slowing down, that may be a good time to change to a cooler environment, at least for a while. Having water available and trusting the mother's intuitions and desires seem to be the most important guiding principles in the use of water in labor. It is important to note that you do not have to have an expensive hot tub/spa already in place. You can simply set up an inexpensive plastic pool, filling it with large kettles of water heated on your stove and/or running a hose from your water heater to the pool. I will comment on each phase of labor and how water may be used in that phase if desired.

You know you are in early/latent labor when the contractions do not feel like they are going away, but increase in intensity and regularity. It becomes difficult to ignore them at this point. If this is your first birth, you may be surprised at the intensity of the contractions early on and wonder if you will be able to make it through the entire process. This is a common feeling, and if you had pre-labor contractions (false labor), you may have already faced this feeling. Elizabeth Davis, midwife, advises birth attendants on what to communicate to a birthing mother in this situation:

> Explain that later on, her body will just take over and work automatically, and she'll find resources for coping that she doesn't even realize she has, if only she'll surrender and let it happen. You might suggest a hot bath for getting used to her sensations.[20]

In regards to the effects of fear on a woman's labor, Michel Odent states,

> Immersion in warm water tends to reduce the level of hormones that we secrete at a high rate when we are cold or frightened. It is well known that a high level of

these hormones, which belong to the adrenalin family, makes the dilation of the cervix take longer; it also becomes more difficult and more dangerous...Thus a bath that is the same temperature as the body protects the mother-to-be against the fight-and-flight response; it achieves the physiological state sometimes called "relaxation response."[21]

It also sometimes occurs in first births that the mother feels the sensations she is having are only cramps or gas, and sometimes by the time she calls her doctor or midwife, or goes to the hospital, she is already fully dilated.

A warm bath in early labor can be just the friendly, reassuring support you need to relax into the journey you are embarking upon. The mental and emotional aspects of yourself really have a chance to surrender to and trust your physiological processes. It can be a time when your mind willingly surrenders to the wisdom of your body. If warm water feels like a helpful element in surrendering to an unknown and seemingly risky endeavor, then by all means, allow its warmth and fluid acceptance to be a catalyst for your own acceptance of the labor process.

Active labor is usually experienced as a shifting of gears into a labor pattern that becomes the dominating force, rather than you being able to change or alter the force of labor with your mind or emotions. Women often enter a tub when they feel this shift occurring, and doing so allows them to relax their body instead of tensing up and resisting. I experienced this change as a quantum leap in what I thought labor would be like and what I thought was possible for me to experience in my body. Once this shift was made, however, I experienced an increased knowingness that the birth really will happen and that my body

(I) can do it. In active labor, contractions become stronger and harder. This can be a very good time for the helpfulness of touch, particularly on the sacrum and shoulders. You will be letting go and sinking deeper into your body and your baby. Upright positions are helpful, as well as standing or walking between contractions. If you have a large tub available to you, you may find that you can flow easily in and out of positions and your partner or doula may find that they can massage you and support your body quite easily. If you have been spending quite a lot of time in early labor in the water, you may find a change of scene to outside the tub or in a different room very helpful. This might provide a time to drain and clean the tub if necessary, as sometimes a little poop comes out as the body opens. Clean fresh water can feel as good as clean fresh sheets on a bed.

Transition from first to second stage, or heavy labor, is from around 7-10 centimeters and is characterized by longer and stronger contractions coming very close together. Women in this phase of labor are usually so centered and in their body that they appear to have little connection to the outside world—an altered state of consciousness that midwives call "laborland," and this is as it should be for this phase of labor. Elizabeth Davis states, "To observe women at this time is a privilege; most have a softness, a rosiness and glow about them as true essence/true nature is revealed. The apparent sleepy, out-of-it quality between contractions is actually an experience of roots, bliss and identification with a force much greater than the individual." [22] If you do enter laborland, no one should try to distract you or pull you out of it, as in that altered state, you have left your rational mind behind and are simply surrendering to letting your body do its work. Sometimes at this stage of labor, women have fears of dying, and indeed women are asked to surrender to such a massive amount of energy streaming through them that it does require a big ego death. This is one reason why, in natural births, women come out of the birth experience stronger and with more confidence and self-esteem than before. They have faced the seemingly impossible and come through it triumphantly.

Some women choose to enter the water for the first time during transition and feel immediate relief. Some women who have already been in the water can't imagine moving elsewhere because the intensity and heaviness are so much greater out of the water. This is why there have been so many accidental water deliveries, because women did not want to move when they were in transition and getting ready to push. If, however, you have been laboring in water for a while, it may feel good to leave the tub and go to the spot where you feel comfortable for the delivery. Dr. Odent has observed, particularly in the home births he has attended, that leaving the warm tub seems to trigger the "fetus ejection reflex." This is the reflex for the delivery of the baby. Frequently, just prior to delivery, women feel frightened, shout out, and have a high level of adrenaline caused by sudden fear. Dr. Odent feels this response may be a natural occurrence that triggers the delivery of the baby, whereas in early labor, fear or intense stress has the opposite effect and slows down the progress of labor.[23]

Your intuition and the guidance of your birth team will help you know where you want to be for the transition into delivery. Often during transition, women have peak experiences as they let go to being more open than they dreamed possible. However, as 10 centimeters is reached, another shift in focus occurs and you become more present in the world for the work of pushing the baby out. The use of water in second stage—delivery of the baby—is described in Chapter 3.

BENEFITS OF WATER LABOR

⬥ The use of water is a "soft" intervention that aids the natural process of labor to occur.

⬥ The use of water in labor in a hospital setting can serve as a bridge between technology and a woman's primal knowledge about the natural process of labor and birth. Water provides an environment of privacy in which the mother can feel her instinctual knowledge about birth and act on that knowledge. Painful vaginal exams and technological interventions are less likely to be performed when the mother is in water, although today there is a type of wireless telemetry (electronic fetal monitoring) that can be used in water. Its use may help the doctor and nurses to feel more comfortable about allowing water labor. If you plan to labor in water in a hospital, it would be wise for you to find out if your hospital has such telemetry available.[24]

⬥ Immersion in a warm bath for labor helps reduce the number of stimuli impinging on the laboring woman, including the stimulus of gravity, and helps the woman focus inwards on her instincts.

⬥ Water offers relief from pain and the intense sensations of labor by relaxing muscles and helping the natural hormonal system for labor to function unimpeded.

⬥ Water allows for freedom of movement and changing of positions, as long as the labor tub is large enough, at least 6 feet in diameter and 2 or so feet deep.

⬥ Water assists labor companions to hold and support the birthing woman more easily than in gravity.

- A large communal pool for labor offers the possibility for sharing your labor with other laboring women, which can be beneficial in certain cases at certain times during labor.

- Water symbolizes relaxation for most people and can be an ever-present reminder to let go and allow the body to do its job.

- Using warm water can help shorten labor.

- Warm water is a way to avoid the use of drugs, which have potentially damaging side effects on the mother and baby. "Where there is a demand for drugs, it is a time to use the water."[25]

- When a woman is pregnant and knows the pool is available, she already has another image of birth, even if she does not use the pool. She can perhaps feel better in advance just knowing the pool is available.[26]

- Water offers a pleasant and soothing environment for the couple to enjoy their labor.

- Water contributes to a sensual atmosphere for birth rather than a more harsh and non-sensual one.

- Water can help a woman make one or more of the necessary emotional and mental shifts from early labor to active labor and then to transition.

- The warmth and fluid acceptance of water can be a catalyst for your own acceptance of the labor process.

- There is no evidence that being in water increases the risk of infections. The vagina is very waterproof. It does not matter if the waters break before entering the pool.[27]

- The use of water in labor is an approach that is now accepted in prestigious teaching hospitals in various high-resource countries. Teaching about the use of laboring in water is an indication that this approach is being accepted by some medical authorities who are responsible for the training of physicians.[28]

RISKS OF WATER LABOR

- If the water in the tub is too hot, or if the woman stays in too long, labor could slow down, and she could have a longer end of first stage.

- If warm water is seen as a hostile environment by the mother, her partner, or members of the birthing team, it is potentially a riskier environment. If the mother feels that *terra firma* is a much more secure environment for her in labor, she needs to act on that feeling rather than what she "thinks" would be an appropriate environment for her.

- There is increased risk when the aim or objective is to deliver the baby in water, rather than water delivery being one possibility. In other words, the more you try to adhere to a preconceived plan rather than being open to the natural flow of your intuition, the more risk there is. In addition, birth attendants need to feel confident in supporting water deliveries when they occur.

PERSONAL STORIES ABOUT WATER AND LABOR

A Mother's Account of Laboring in Water

by Robbie Davis-Floyd [29]

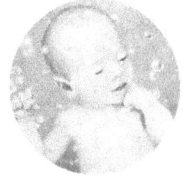

I have given birth twice: the first time to a daughter by cesarean section in the hospital, the second time to a son by vaginal birth in my home. The two experiences are as different as dark and light, day and night, but the lesson that I learned from each experience was the same: to trust myself and what I know.

There were things that I knew this second time, and that, unlike the first time, I trusted—that the boy was a baby (he was); that he would weigh exactly 10 pounds (he did); that my labor would be three days long (it was); and that I would need a totally supportive environment which included warm water to get through it (I did).

In early labor I paced around the grocery store, peering at tomatoes and secretly hoping that something dramatic would happen—like my waters breaking at the checkout counter. But, to my great disappointment, no one even noticed that I was in labor. I returned home to the rhythmic ringing of hammers on wood— my husband Robert and several of his friends were climbing around on top of the temporary room they had constructed around the rented hot tub, which we had placed on our cement porch just outside our front door. I couldn't believe my eyes—in the time I had been gone, they had practically finished the room! Double sheets of plastic had been nailed across the wooden supports to serve as walls, which had been further insulated with almost every blanket and quilt in the house, including some made by my great-grandmother. Truly, my husband had constructed a "womb room" for me—his labor had prepared a special space for mine. Although it was the dead of winter—19 degrees outside—with all those blankets on the walls, and the space heater going, that room stayed as warm as a real womb for three days!

Around 10 pm, the midwives came and checked me, and unpacked their bags and went to bed. They said, "Don't get in a hurry! This is going to take a long time—you're not even in real labor yet. You're only four centimeters!" That scared me because I got stuck at four centimeters in my first birth and ended up with a cesarean. So, around midnight, looking for some comfort and reassurance, I got into the bathtub (the hot tub wasn't ready) and stayed there in the warm water, with Rima rubbing my back, for a long time.

The midwives got up periodically to take turns sitting with me while I stayed in the bathtub. They told me, over and over, not to get my expectations up because I still wasn't in real labor. Cathy said, "Honey, I know it hurts, I know it feels to you like real labor, but these contractions are just very early ones. They are going to have to get a lot longer, a lot stronger, and a lot closer together before you're going to be in real labor."

I didn't really believe her, because the contractions were just like the ones I had felt the first time, and the nurses hadn't said anything about them being "early labor." It wasn't until Day 3 that I finally understood the difference.

By 3:00 a.m., everyone in the house was asleep but me. I had dried off and climbed into bed to snuggle with Robert. He dozed off blissfully, but I lay awake and breathed through contractions all night. Around 7 a.m., our friend Phillip, who was there because he knew he would never have a child and really wanted to witness a birth, came and told me that the hot tub was ready. It had taken hours to fill, because we hadn't installed a water circulation system of any kind (we had been able to find a used hot tub for only $300, but the machinery to hook it up was too expensive for us). Phillip and Robert were having to fill it with a hose connected to the hot water heater, which could only produce enough hot water to run for a few minutes at a time. So, Phillip had been heroically augmenting this by heating huge kettles full of water on the stove, and then carrying them to the womb room and dumping them in. He presided over that kettle-laden stove for three days; his labor too was an essential ingredient in mine.

I was thrilled that the tub I had wanted to labor in so much was finally ready. I have always felt most blissful floating in water or soaking in a hot shower, and most peaceful looking at water, whether in oceans, lakes, rivers, or swimming pools. Like Rima, I swam throughout my pregnancies—the pool was the only place where I felt weightless, totally supported by my environment. I slipped eagerly out of bed without waking Robert and, in the middle of a contraction, sank into my hot tub's celestial blue welcoming warmth, feeling just like Eve in Eden (see Figure 2.5). The water inside and the water outside of me seemed as one.

The morning of the second day of labor, the midwives got me out of the tub to check my dilation. I was "still four centimeters," so they told me to call them when the contractions got stronger, and went home to take care of their children! I got back in the tub, and stayed there most of the morning.

I spent hours that day having contractions in the tub's warmth— I even ate lunch in there. Robert had thoughtfully built a little platform off the side of the tub to put things on, so I could eat and drink without having to leave the tub's comfort. I remember the taste of that food to this day, and the overwhelming awareness of how much my body needed that nourishment.

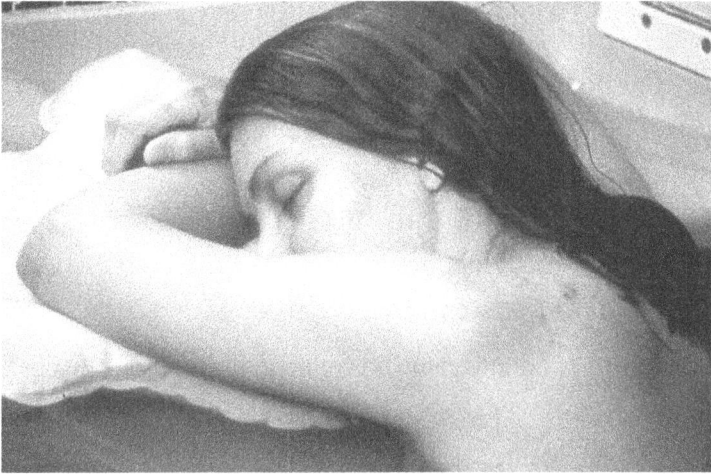

Figure 2.5. *Robbie as "Eve in Eden" in "laborland" in her hot tub. Photo by Peter Gonzalez, used with permission.*

After noon, my contractions began to space out more and more, until finally around 2:00 p.m. (about the time I was waiting for the OB to come back from church to do the cesarean in my first birth), the contractions stopped altogether. I was out of the tub and dressed by now, and I was shaking with fear because I didn't know what was going to happen or how to deal with it. I told Rima that I wanted her to do something to make me feel better. I trusted her so completely—I felt that it was within her power to help me release this paralyzing fear that I wouldn't make it, and would end up in the hospital with another cesarean. So, Rima helped me create a ritual.

We put a bunch of tall candles on the floor and everyone there made a circle around them. At Rima's suggestion, we started stating our fears one by one, and then throwing them into the flames to symbolically release them. I found myself relaxing and feeling more unselfconscious and natural in performing the ritual. The ritual was very cathartic, especially for me, because one of the fears I had was that I couldn't communicate with Robert, that he would think I was being ridiculous during labor and wouldn't support me. But when he started doing the ritual like everyone else, and stating his own fears, I felt a sudden rush of openness between us, and after the ritual was over I went to him crying and he really opened up to me and held me for a long time, just standing there in the living room in our magic circle.

After that, I suddenly realized that the hour when the cesarean had happened four years ago was long past, and that I had finally entered completely uncharted territory. I was free! The past pattern no longer had the power to map itself onto my present experience! My relief was overwhelming.

I got into bed to rest and soon the contractions began again, coming about every 10 minutes. They stayed at that rate all that night, so I was even able to sleep quite well for about four or five hours.

On the third day a contraction awoke me at dawn. I felt tremendously refreshed and extremely grateful for such a wonderful sleep. The contractions were still coming every 10 minutes, so I ate a good breakfast and got back into the tub, which Phillip had managed to keep warm for me overnight. Soon the contractions picked up in intensity. By noon they were coming three minutes apart, and I was in serious distress, truly stunned by the strength and power of the contractions. The midwives came back, unpacked, and checked me, and announced with great glee that I was now 6 centimeters! I was furious. The exam had been worse than the contractions, and I couldn't believe that an entire morning of such contractions had resulted in no more than 2 cm. of progress. But the midwives were elated and they said, "Now, you're really in labor!"

By mid-afternoon I was arching my back in the tub during contractions, pulling on Robert's arms and pushing against the side of the tub with my feet (see Figure 2.6).

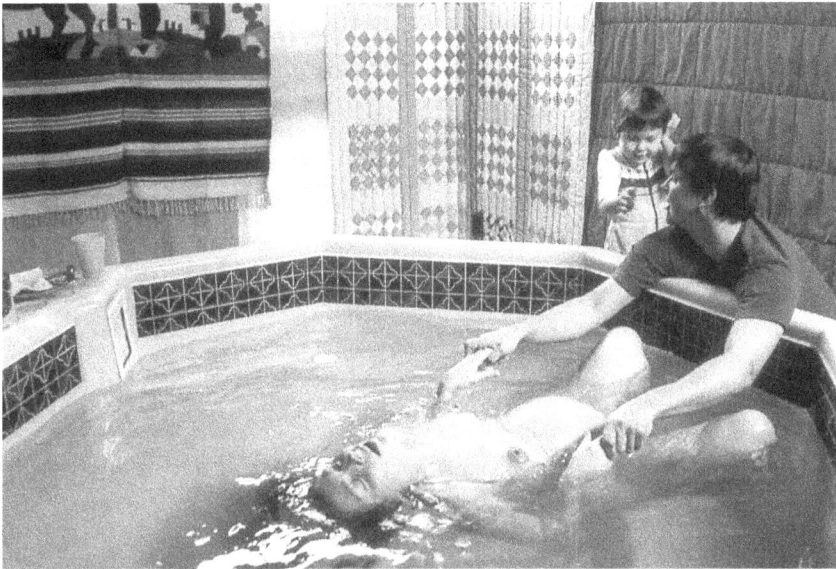

Figure 2.6. *Robbie in the tub in heavy, active labor using her husband's arms to pull against and with her 4-year-old daughter Peyton watching. Photo by Peter Gonzalez, used with permission.*

It was the only way I could stand the pain without going nuts. The contractions felt like one person was stabbing me in the stomach with a knife and twisting it, while another person was stabbing me in the back with a long sword and pushing on it. The pain was so overwhelming that I vowed I would never again harshly judge a woman for asking for an epidural or other drugs to avoid feeling such pain. I "got it" that you have to be completely committed to taking the experience as it comes. Most of us in the US are used to some degree of control over our physical sensations, so I found it valuable to fully experience a physical reality without such control—but I could certainly understand why many women would not desire that sort of experience. There were many moments during that labor when, if somebody had offered me rescue—a quick way to get out of my body, I would have taken it! I found myself repeatedly envisioning a window in the sky. I kept thinking, "If I could just step through that window, I'd be in Tahiti." Later Jane English (who wrote a book called *Different Doorway: Adventures of a Cesarean Born*, about her experiences with remembering her own cesarean birth) told me that the "window in the sky" was my programming from my birth by cesarean in 1951, in which I had indeed been "rescued" through such a window!

In the midst of such pain as I would never have believed I could survive, I began making chanting sounds. Often my 4-year-old daughter Peyton would chant with Robert and me during contractions. We chanted for hours, and I was truly impressed by how much of the pain could be channeled through me and out by a powerful sound.

At one point everyone else in attendance—8 people in total, including Phillip, our photographer Peter Gonzalez, my midwives Cathy and Debbie, my doula Rima, and her young daughter Mela—came in, encircled the hot tub, and began chanting along with us. My contractions were in synchrony, stronger than ever, and I chanted my pain and my joy at our precious harmony, and the womb room sounded and resounded like a Catholic cathedral.

After an hour or so more, I had to get out of the tub to go to the bathroom. When I finished, I noticed that the bed had been freshly made up with my favorite sheets and quilt to receive my newborn and me. It looked so inviting! I dove onto it in the middle of a contraction, and suddenly everything changed. Without any pre-plan, I simply gave up and surrendered to the overwhelming force of the contractions. Until that moment, I had been struggling to maintain myself as separate from the pain—to sing, dance, float, or chant with it, while still maintaining myself as separate from it. Suddenly I just let that effort go, and I said to the pain, "Take me, I'm yours." Then a miracle happened. I felt that I, body and soul, became the pain, and once there was no more separation between me and the pain, there was no more pain! I lay there on the bed, utterly relaxed, breathing softly, in total peace. I could hear the midwives whispering "Good, that's really good." And that was, for me, one of the most important life-lessons of the birth—the value of yielding, of complete surrender.

And then, just as suddenly, I came out of what I now know was "laborland." Unaware that I was in transition, feeling only that with each contraction I would surely fly through the roof or leap through the window, I was truly amazed that the house did not simply explode as a result of this tremendous force inside of me. I crouched on the bed in terror and panic and panted to Robert that I could not do it, that I thought I would die. His strong hands grasped my shoulders, and his calm voice soothed me.

Suddenly I heard Rima, who had been rubbing my back, exclaim, "Oh my!" and I felt her stand up. My waters, intact until that moment, had broken and anointed both Rima and my best quilt. Truly, there was water everywhere with this birth! Rima didn't seem to mind, and the midwives laughed. How different from the hospital, where any liquids I exuded onto the birthing suite's Halston sheets were greeted with much clucking and headshaking and immediately cleaned up.

Around 6:30 pm, the midwives checked my dilation again. I couldn't believe my ears. They said, "Robbie, you're 10 centimeters! Where do you want to be to have your baby?" "In the hot tub," I exclaimed, astonished that I was really going to have my baby. I don't remember getting there—the next thing I knew, Robert, swimsuit-clad, was sitting on the molded seat inside the tub, while I, naked, crouched on his knees and tried to find a good position for pushing.

Now I have to tell you something that is very personal, but I am going to include it here because it was wonderful, and if you know that I did it, maybe that will give you the license you need to break a few social rules and have this pleasure too. In spite of the fact that our hot tub was surrounded by people, and that Cathy in her bathing suit was right in there with us, I turned facing Robert and I whispered in his ear, "Please rub my clit!" The energy that I was feeling was intense, and accompanying the intense pain of the contractions was an equally intense sexual desire. In the hospital, he wouldn't even get in the shower with me, but here in our own home, he overcame his embarrassment and complied with my request. Very quickly, I had an incredible orgasm. It was an island of ecstasy in the midst of an ocean of pain. I was sure that if I ever give birth again (which I didn't), I would be wanting to do a lot more of that sort of thing, and I would make sure that Robert and I had the privacy for labor that would enhance the passionate nature of the birth experience. (This was long before Debra Pascali-Bonaro's production of the wonderful film *Orgasmic Birth*, so at the time, I felt that this was the best-kept secret—that labor and birth are inherently sexual processes and can benefit from nipple and clitoral stimulation during labor. After all, it is the same natural hormone—oxytocin—that flows through our bodies during sex, labor, birth, and breastfeeding.)

I settled on squatting in the water between Robert's knees, and I pushed during contractions while everyone chanted, but I didn't put my heart and soul into it because the pushing hurt more than the contractions alone, and I was disappointed because I had been told it would likely hurt less. About 20 minutes into the pushing, Cathy got very nervous because the baby's heart tones were dropping, and I heard her mutter under her breath something about going to the hospital if they got any lower. I looked at her through the haze of pain and energy required for pushing, and my entire body suddenly flooded with the absolute certainty that *my baby was fine. I knew* there was no danger. I leaned forward and opened my mouth to communicate the wonder and the certainty of this knowing to my midwife, but another contraction seized me in its bony grip, and I was unable to speak. So Cathy, still nervous, asked me to get out of the tub and push on the toilet. She felt that the baby was stuck on the Ischeal spines and was worried that his oxygen supply might be compromised. I complied.

I do not regret the experience of getting out of the tub, even though I had planned to give birth in the water, because the second most important lesson of the birth happened to me as I ran down the hall to the bathroom. The walls of the hall, and all the other people running down it with me, suddenly fell away, and I was completely alone in a universe of my own making. I *got it* that this time there would be no rescue. There was no window in the sky to take me to Tahiti. There was no white knight in shining armor to rescue me from the dragon of pain. No one and no thing could do this for me. It was totally and completely up to me. Until then, most things in my life had come easy to me—being first in my class in high school was a breeze, as was graduating *Summa cum Laude* from my university. I had never had to work really hard at anything. And so, unconsciously,

I had set it all up so that it would come to this existential moment of realization that I had to do this thing. The only way out of it was through it, and *I* had to do it.

And then I was, finally and for the first time, truly ready to give birth. My commitment at long last was complete. I shivered with the realization that *this was it*. Now, here, me in this place, feeling this pain—no, *doing* this pain. I was actively doing the pain to myself now—no more avoidance. I was leaning back against the toilet lid, with my feet propped up high on colorful Mexican baskets. I put my heart and soul, and every muscle in my body, into pushing the baby past the Ischial spines—the "stuck place," as the midwives called it. The pain was unbelievable, but it was tempered by my new-found determination. I was going to do this thing, no matter how much it hurt. There was tremendous relief in that commitment.

There was also relief in my subsequent discovery, at long last, of *how* to push. I had been straining the wrong muscles, and I finally figured out that if I bore down from my diaphragm, I could actually gauge the proper angle to push from and into. After that my pushes became much more effective

After 20 minutes of pushing on the toilet, the midwives announced that the baby was past the "stuck place," and his heart-rate was back up. I accepted being on the toilet as useful at the time, but I was not at all happy about it. So, I was very relieved to get out of that ignominious position.

It's strange—even though my official plan had been to give birth in the water, I knew from the beginning that I was not actually going to do that. I knew that I needed the water for labor, but my bed has always been my "safe place." When I got up from the toilet, I instinctively headed for the bed. Robert piled on first, with his back to the wall, and I got between his legs, semi-upright, leaning against him, and then side-lying (see Figures 2.7 and

2.8). It took me then about 50 minutes to push out my baby. I have tried but I cannot describe the overwhelming relief and release I experienced when the baby suddenly flew out. I sank back into Robert's arms, carrying with me the impression of my newborn lying on the bed, asleep and breathing well—so peaceful. I just wanted to stare at him in amazement.

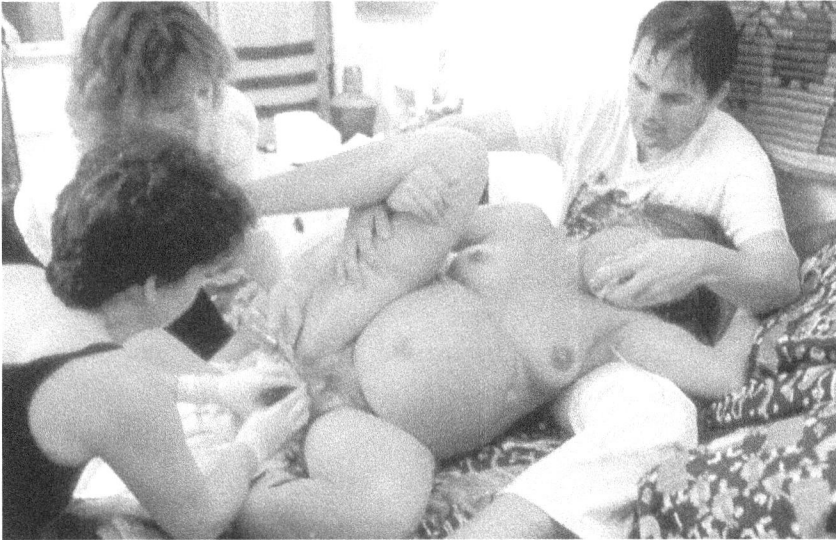

Figure 2.7. *Robbie about to give birth in bed. As her birth facilitator/doula, I was on the other side of the bed, allowing the midwives, Cathy and Debbie, space to deal with the brief shoulder dystocia her baby experienced. Yes, upright positions for birth are best, but when you have been up and moving around a lot during labor, it does not matter if you lie down for the moments of birth, and side-lying is better than on your back as it allows more pelvic space. Note the oxygen mask Robbie's husband Robert is holding over her face at the midwives' suggestion. She found that to be an extremely empowering use of technology, as the pure oxygen gave her added energy just when she needed it most! Photo by Peter Gonzalez, used with permission.*

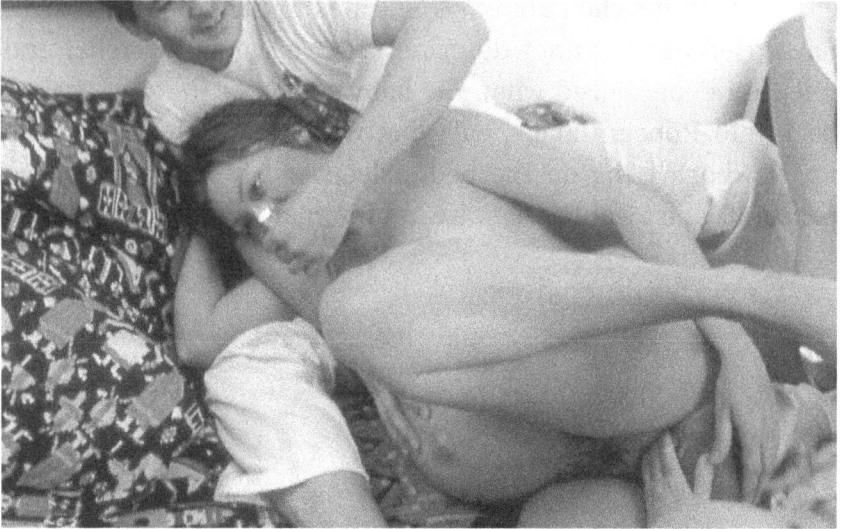

Figure 2.8. *The baby's head is out, and Robbie cradles it in her hand. She said, "That feeling is forever imprinted in my hand's palm and my heart's memory." Photo by Peter Gonzales, used with permission.*

But the midwives were in a hurry for me to hold and nurse Jason, and he started crying. After about half an hour of their fussing, having me try one nipple and then the other, one position and then another, Jason was still crying, and I finally asked everyone to leave so that I could hear the baby. Then I held Jason up in front of me and silently asked him what he needed (Figure 2.8).

Instantly I sensed from him that he needed to be in the water. I asked our photographer Peter to fill up the baby bathtub with warm tap water and put it on the bed. As soon as Robert and I lowered Jason into the tub, he stretched out his little body to its fullest extension, opened his eyes and looked at us, pulled my finger into his mouth and sucked it vigorously, and then suddenly went limp in the water in total relaxation, all his tension gone (Figure 2.9). He has been an extremely mellow child ever since, even-tempered and easy to soothe.

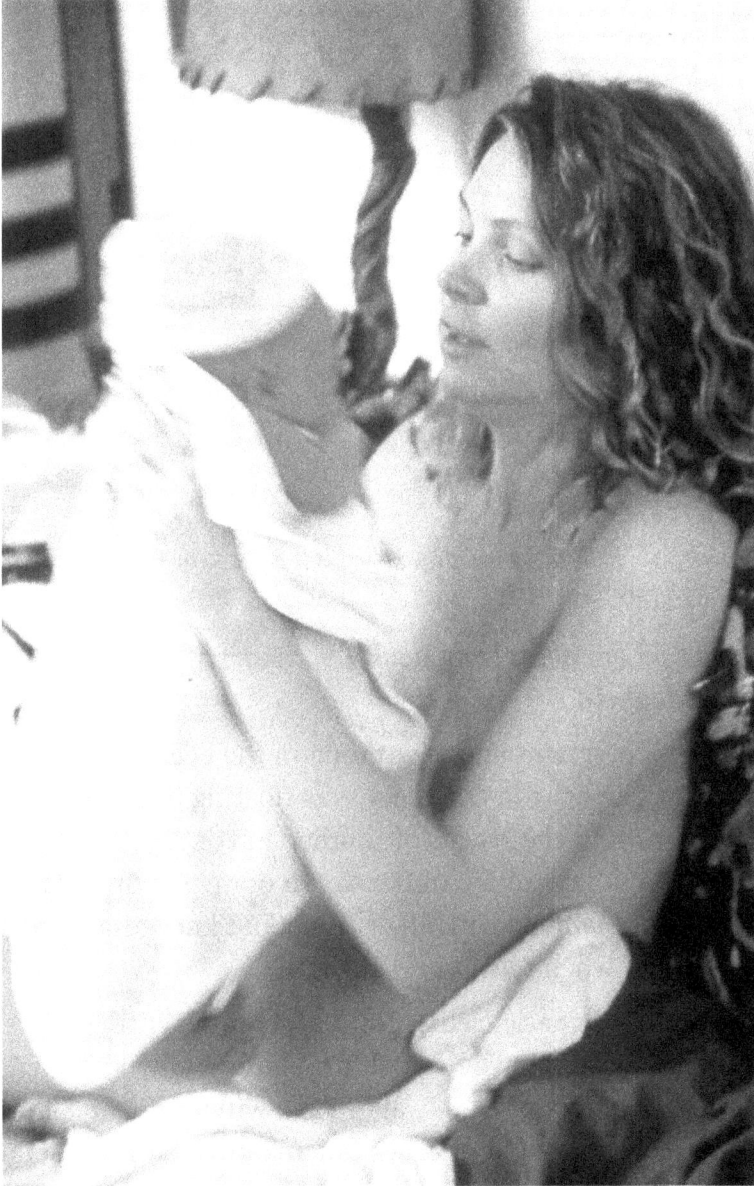

Figure 2.9. *Robbie silently asking Jason what he needed. Photo by Peter Gonzalez, used with permission.*

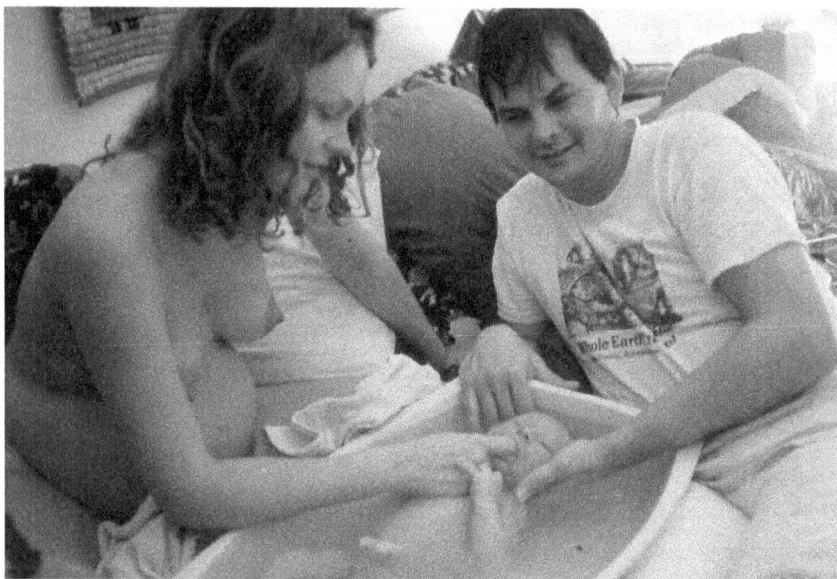

Figure 2.10. *Baby Jason mellows out in his tub. Photo by Peter Gonzalez, used with permission.*

Subsequent Comments from Robbie Six Years after Jason's 1984 Birth

When I was pregnant and swimming in the ocean, I remember feeling that the baby inside of me was floating in my ocean and I was floating in the ocean of Mother Earth. The baby in my womb was a mirror of me in the womb of my Earth Mother. At that moment I felt one with all of creation. I knew that I wanted to be in water when I went into labor.

All in all, I experienced around 20 hours laboring in water. I wonder if I would have been able to successfully give birth at home if I had not labored in water. I'm a wimp when it comes to pain. Yet I did not want analgesia of any kind, so I felt I would need whatever my environment could give me in the way of labor support. I believed water would support me in labor. If I could do anything to help me relax and get through what I expected to be a long labor, it would be to immerse myself in warm water. Our small bathtub was pretty unsatisfactory. When the hot tub was finally ready, I felt so nurtured sinking into the warm water. The pain of the contractions was still there but all around me was bliss. My pain was surrounded by lots and lots of warm pleasure. I felt like the water was an ally and a friend, a protector. To be in the hot tub was to be in my own private space. Now, in retrospect, I realize that I had too many people at my birth, too much observation of me. If I did it over again, I'd have fewer people there. Being in the water was about as private as I got during Jason's birth. When I felt intense, dagger-like pain and was in the hot tub, I felt like my body was big enough to handle my pain because I was in the bigger space of the hot tub. During earlier labor, I didn't want anyone else in there with me. I wanted them on the outside. Robert would hold my hands and I would stretch back in the tub, as shown in the photo above, but I didn't want anyone else in my space. It was a big labor, a big pain, and I needed a big space.

Not having gravity in water, being able to float and be light made me lighter with the pain. I felt like the pain would come in through and my back and my stomach and be channeled electro-magnetically out of my mouth as I chanted. Because I was in water, I was able to become an electro-magnetic current for transmitting the energy out through me. The pain was an electrical current and when I was in water, I could conduct that current right through me and out through my mouth through chanting. When I was out of the tub, I don't remember being able to do that. It was more like I had to *contain* the pain when I was out of the tub. Often when I was out of the tub, I thought I was going to split apart because of the enormity of the contractions. When I was in the tub, I felt I could *channel* the pain and release it. I felt that my primary support "person" besides my husband was the water and the tub. Without the water, I might well have ended up screaming for drugs and going to the hospital. The water was bliss all around me. The pain and the bliss were like a counterbalance for each other.

In my case, the tub was really dirty when delivery time came near, because some poop had come out and was floating in the water in little pieces. I think in my ideal vision, I would have another clean tub to get in to deliver the baby (or I wish we could have afforded to actually install our hot tub properly so it could be drained and cleaned for delivery). I think going from one tub to another could have triggered the "fetus ejection reflex" Michel Odent talks about and the clean tub would have been very comfortable for delivery of the baby and to relax and bond with him after he was out.

Even though it was freezing cold outside, I could stay completely warm by having a towel over the part of my body that stuck out of the water. People would pour warm water all over me each time they brought warm water from the kitchen—that was intensely blissful! Also, when they would bring the hose and run more hot water from the water heater into the tub, I would feel incredibly nurtured. I would get this infusion of warmth that would pervade my whole body and spread all over me. I would relax into that warmth and it was fabulous to experience that bliss along with the pain of the contractions. That's what made the pain bearable and taught me I could experience bliss at the same time as intense pain. Perhaps if I had given birth again, I would have been more able to experience the bliss and the pain as one, as I did for that short time I described above.

A Birth Attendant's Story:
Rima as Birth Facilitator/Doula
for Jason's Labor and Birth

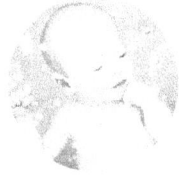

As Birth Facilitator for Jason's birth, I knew I would have a healing time for myself as well as supporting them in their process. Robbie and I had much in common. We were both born by cesarean. We were both only children, growing up within 30 miles of each other. We were both keenly interested in pre- and perinatal psychology. I was two months pregnant at the time with my second daughter Orien. For a long time, Orien and Jason were in the same classroom and are still great friends. I often wonder how much Orien learned and healed from being at Jason's birth while inside my womb.

From my own memories of being born cesarean, and from birthing my first daughter, Mela, vaginally, I knew that coming out the vagina is a foreign concept to a cesarean-born person. Therefore, I worked with Robbie to create and integrate an image for the possibility of a vaginal delivery. Not having had that possibility as a kinesthetic reality in our own physiologies meant taking the time and energy to make that possibility a reality for the births of our children. Since neither of us had experienced the methodical flow of contractions and the intense sensations accompanying them during our own births, we were both new at learning what labor was like. Water was a key element and symbol for Robbie and for me, allowing us to feel the safety we needed in order to go forward with vaginal births.

I see from Robbie's birth and from what I know now about water being a symbol for the feminine, the Mother, that water was that receptive, feminine force that could receive Robbie and be a space within which she felt secure and able to let the energy of the birth move through her. The midwives in attendance were not as able as the water to be such an unconditional feminine force. I see the potential for water being used in hospital settings to provide women with the kind of feminine support they need to deliver their babies without needless interventions. The possibility exists that water can provide what may be lacking in some of the birth attendants—that kind of feminine receptivity that will allow women to birth naturally. Using water for labor is kind of like introducing a doula—a caring, unconditional, and receptive woman—to the birth environment. Her job is not to disrupt labor but to facilitate it to occur naturally. If a hospital, doctor, or midwife is at least willing to allow women to get in water for some amount of time during labor or delivery, they could drastically reduce the number of interventions and interruptions in the birth process.

The room that Robert created for Jason's birth was truly a private, receptive space, just big enough for the large hot tub and occasional people and things around the edges. It was possible to feel serenity and solitude in that room, even though the two midwives in attendance were bustling around and discussing various things in the other parts of the house. That room was definitely Robbie's space for labor.

Since she had been swimming throughout her pregnancy, Robbie was already conditioned to "swim" through her labor. The tub was large enough that she could move in all directions at once if she wanted to and when she had contractions, that is often what she did. Sometimes she would spiral around in the water with a contraction while making deep guttural chanting sounds, much like I would imagine our friends the dolphins and whales do when they are in labor. One of her favorite positions during a contraction was to float on her back, knees bent and feet against the side of the tub. As shown in the photo, Robert would hold both of her hands while he was standing or kneeling at the tub's rim. When she had a contraction, she would push her body straight out and as the energy subsided, she would relax her knees. She was also able to doze and even sleep in the hot tub by floating her head on an inflatable pillow. She was a Goddess giving birth. Water was her safe haven and I could feel that she would definitely be able to birth Jason vaginally. She allowed the water to be her friend and confidante and to receive her pain and uncertainties, helping her to be as fluid about them as the water. Just knowing that Robert or I were nearby to hold her hand or sing or chant with her seemed to be enough. When it came time to deliver Jason, she went from the tub to the bathroom to her bed, and received her 10-pound son with Robert holding her in his arms, the midwives in position, and her daughter Peyton and my daughter Mela watching eagerly (see Figures 2.11, 2.12, and 2.13).

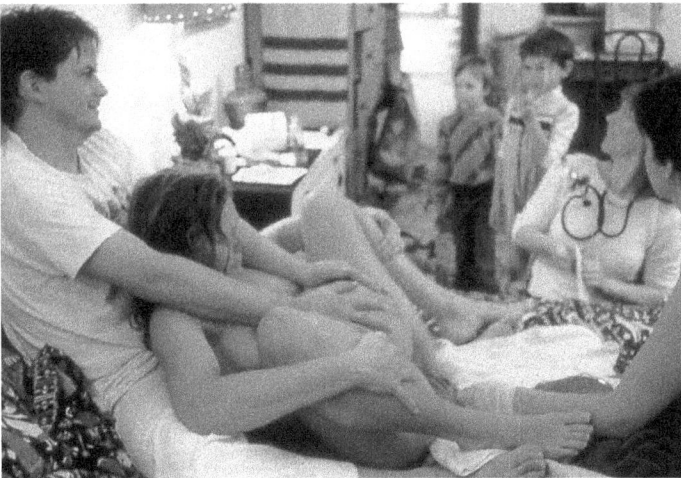

Figure 2.11. *Robbie birthing Jason with Peyton (right) and Mela (left) watching. At one point, Peyton dragged in a high bar stool so she could sit on it and have a better view. Photo by Peter Gonzalez, used with permission.*

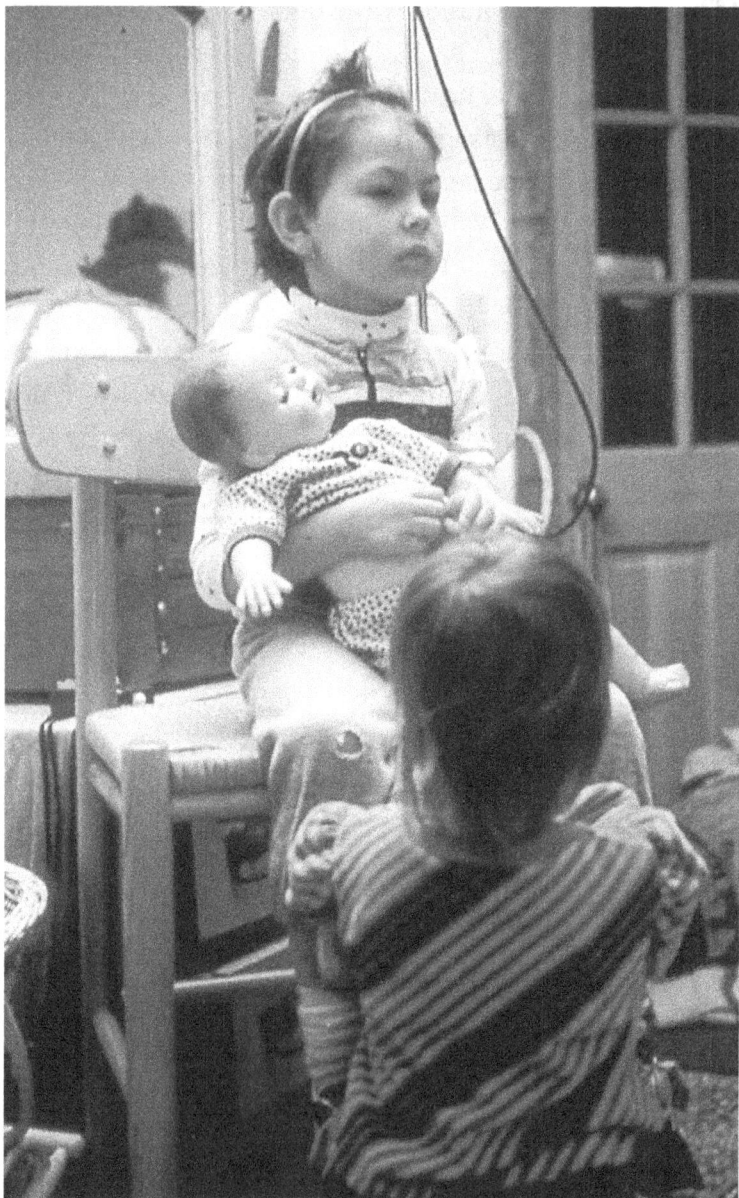

Figure 2.12. *Peyton sitting on her bar stool, clutching a boy doll—for Robbie had intuitively known the baby would be a boy—with Mela about to climb up to join her. Photo by Peter Gonzalez, used with permission.*

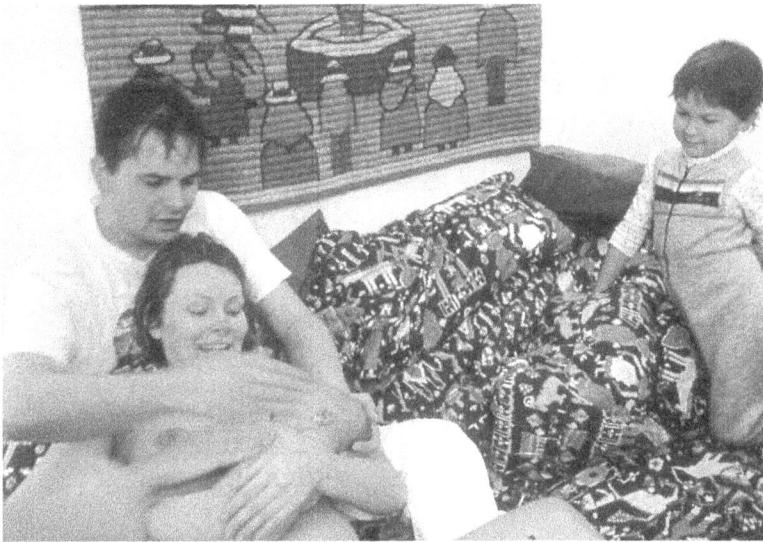

Figure 2.13. *The newborn family, as Peyton approaches to meet her new brother. But first, she had taken a good look at Robbie's vagina, as, even though she had watched the whole birth, she was still astonished that something so big could come through something so small! Photo by Peter Gonzalez, used with permission.*

A Birth Attendant's Story: Michel Odent

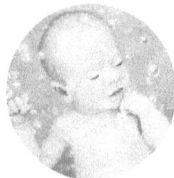

Quoted from His Book *Water and Sexuality*

A woman, living locally in the heart of the town, had never before been in a swimming pool; she could not swim and used to claim that she would have nothing to do with such tricks. However, on the day of the birth, she was irresistibly attracted by the water and could not leave the bath before the birth of her baby.

If a mother-to-be goes to the bath before the onset of hard labour, the contractions may stop. On the other hand, the cervix may dilate several centimeters quite rapidly. However, this will not necessarily prevent the protraction of the later stages of labour. Alternatively, if the mother-to-be gets into the water only when hard labour is established and when the dilation of the cervix is well advanced (for example, at least 6 centimeters), the end of the first stage can be very fast; in the region of one hour for a first baby.

On entering the pool, the mother often gives a great sigh, expressing relief and even well-being. After that, rapid dilation is often accompanied by what might be called a deep regression. She cuts herself off from our world, forgetting what she has learned, what she has read, all her received ideas. She dares to shout out without restraint, and loses control of her breathing and position. Well-intentioned attendants should become less and less intrusive, as her inner trip [into what midwives call "laborland"] takes her deeper and deeper. It is as if the water were protecting her from useless stimuli.

If the midwife is familiar with birth in an atmosphere of intimacy and spontaneity, she has no need to disturb the birth process with vaginal examinations. Even from the next room she will know what is happening: she has only to listen. She can assess the stage of labour according to how fast, how deeply and how noisily the woman is breathing. The midwife can also sense when the labour has stopped and when the contractions are no longer efficient. It often means that the baby is not far away.

This is because during this time—a period that Sheila Kitzinger called "Rest and Be Thankful," the uterus is regrouping itself around the newly descended baby. This process can take up to 30 minutes.

A Baby's Perspective on Labor in Water as Imagined by Rima Star

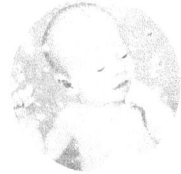

My Mom had been swimming with me inside of her all through my pregnancy. I was born at the end of the summer and many times I heard Mom tell people the water helped her cool off. She said it helped me cool off too because she was "baking" me inside! I liked my Mom. She would laugh a lot when we had our time in the water.

When the little hormonal buzzer sounded and the action of labor started, I began to wonder if we were going to have fun doing this or not. The energy felt really powerful and I could tell that my comfortable life inside my mother was going to change in a big way. I knew this had to happen eventually, but I was wondering if the "getting there" was going to be alright or not.

Then I heard my mother's voice and she said, "Oh, I'm so excited, I'm going to be holding you in my arms before long!"

That sounded really good to me too and I decided we could do this thing called "labor" together. I relaxed in my body and let myself feel the uterus hugging me and helping me to my new destination.

I heard my Dad's voice asking Mom if she wanted him to get our big hot tub clean and filled with water. She said, "That would be nice." While he was doing that, she got up and moved around, walking and swaying to some music she had put on. That felt really good and the hugs of the uterus began coming closer and closer together. I heard her say, "Baby, we can do this. It's safe to come out." I always felt so good when she would talk directly to me. I felt more excitement and more energy.

Next thing I knew, she had gone to the bathroom and flushed the toilet. That was always an interesting sound to me. This time I had the feeling that I was the one that would be swirling down and out like the sound of the water I heard.

She turned on the shower and stood under it, singing a lullaby. She really relaxed when the water was rolling over her, and as she relaxed I felt my head move even further against the cervix of her body. "Wow! This is it," I thought. She left the shower and walked around outside. She said it was a beautiful night but soon the sun would be coming up. I wondered what it would be like to see sun like she saw it.

Soon my father came outside and told her the tub was ready. She was really glad because the energy waves of contractions were building even more. She sank into the big tub and I felt her whole body relax even more. Then I forgot to even think about what was happening and she did too and it felt like we were swimming and swimming with the energy contractions. She would yell out and make sounds and I would yell out too.

At a certain point when I felt my head move through the cervix, she yelled out and suddenly left the tub, saying she wanted to be on the ground. I felt like I was about to drop out. She squatted on the grass with my dad holding her from behind and began grunting and groaning with me moving through her tunnel. The waters that had been sheltering my head burst and I could feel the cool air on the top of my head. A few more grunts and groans and contractions and my head was out, then my shoulders and whole body. I could feel the softness and coolness of the green grass and opened my eyes and there she was! I smiled as she picked me up and held me in her warm arms. Soon my Dad had a blanket around both of us and I could actually see the rays of pink light in the morning sky. "We did it, Mom," I said silently, beaming up at her. "What a glorious day to be born!"

Endnotes

1 *Webster's Ninth New Collegiate Dictionary*, Springfield, Massachusetts, Merriam-Webster, Inc. 1983, p.

2 Gaskin, Ina May, *Spiritual Midwifery*, Summertown, Tn.: The Book Publishing Co., 1978, p.340.

3 For a description of "the holistic model of birth and health care," which encompasses and unites body, mind, and spirit, see Davis-Floyd, Robbie (2018). "The Technocratic, Humanistic, and Holistic Paradigms of Birth and Health Care," in *Ways of Knowing about Birth: Mothers, Midwives, Medicine, and Birth Activism*. Long Grove IL: Waveland Press, pp. 3-44.

4 Odent, Michel, "The Fetus Ejection Reflex," *Birth: Issues in Perinatal Care* 14(2),1987, pp.104-105.

5 Cunningham et al., *Williams Obstetrics*, 25th edition, 2018, p. 410.

6 Davis-Floyd, Robbie, Michel Odent, personal conversation, Oct. 29, 1990, Austin, Tx.

7 Davis-Floyd, Robbie, *Birth as an American Rite of Passage*, 3rd edition, Abingdon, Oxon, UK: Routledge, 2022.

8 See Alfirevic Z, GML Gyte, A Cuthbert, D Devane. 2017. "Continuous Cardiotocography as a Form of Electronic Fetal Monitoring for Fetal Assessment During Labour." *Cochrane Database of Systematic Reviews* 2. doi.org/doi:10.1002/14651858.CD006066.pub3

9 Michel Odent, Austin Lecture, October 29, 1990.

10 Davis-Floyd, Robbie. *Birth as an American Rite of Passage*, 3rd edition. Abingdon, Oxon: Routledge, 2022.

11 Odent, Michel, *Water and Sexuality*, New York: Viking Penguin, 1990, p.2.

12 Peterson, Gayle, *Birthing Normally: A Personal Growth Approach to Childbirth*, 1981, p.4

13 See Cheyney, Melissa, and Robbie Davis-Floyd. "Birth and the Big Bad Wolf: Biocultural Evolution and Human Childbirth." In *Birthing Techno-Sapiens: Human-Technology Co-Evolution and the Future of Reproduction*. London: Routledge 2021, pp. 15-46.

14 WHO Human Reproduction Programme. 2015. "Who Statement on Caesarean Section Rates." *Reproductive Health Matters* 23 (45): 149.

15 See Anim-Somual M, RMD Smyth, AM Cyna, A Cuthbert. 2018. "Epidural versus Non-Epidural or No Analgesia for Pain Management in Labour." *Cochrane Databaase of Systematic Reviews* 5. CD000331. doi:10 1002/14651858 and McKoy K. 2017. "Epidural Side-Effects." Found at: https://draxe.com/health/epidural-side-effects/.

16 Odent, *Water and Sexuality*, p.5.

17 Quoted on p. 170 of Church, Linda K. 1989. "Water Birth: One Birthing Center's Observations," *Journal of Nurse-Midwifery* 34(4):165-170. https://doi.org/10.1016/0091-2182(89) 90076-1.

18 Odent, *Water and Sexuality*, p.1.

19 Odent, *Water and Sexuality*, p. 12-13

20 Davis, Elizabeth, *Heart and Hands: A Guide to Midwifery*. Santa Fe: John Muir Publications, 1981, p.94.

21 Odent, *Water and Sexuality*, p.5.

22 Davis, *Heart and Hands*, p.99.

23 Odent, Austin Lecture, October, 1990.

24 Kara, Kelly and Suzanne Miller. "Water as a Technology to Support Embodied Autonomous Birthing." In *Birthing Techno-Sapiens: Human-Technology Co-Evolution and the Future of Reproduction*, edited by Robbie Davis-Floyd. London: Routledge, 2021, pp. 179-182.

25 Odent, Interview, October 30, 1990, Austin, Tx.,

26 Odent, Interview, Oct. 30, 1990, Austin, Tx.

27 Odent, Interview, Oct. 30, 1990, Austin, Tx.

28 Odent, Interview, Oct. 30, 1990, Austin, Tx.

29 This story is excerpted from Davis-Floyd, Robbie, *"Knowing: A Story of Two Births,"* unpublished manuscript, 2000.

Chapter 3

WATER DELIVERY

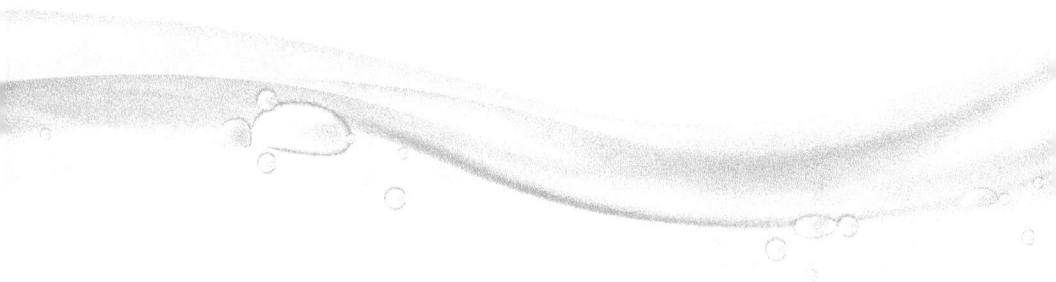

THE IMPORTANCE OF YOUR BIRTHING ENVIRONMENT

Environments are extremely important anytime, but particularly in birth. During childbirth, your perception may be nonlinear and open. You may tend to experience your environment as an extension of yourself rather than as separate from you. You may be more likely to remember a cool wind on your back and how it made you feel than you would remember who opened a window or door and why. Many women have told me the entire room felt like it was expanding as their cervix or perineum opened or felt like it was contracting as movement pushed against a resistant opening. The inner and outer worlds tend to become one in a real way for the birthing mother and baby.

Often, your birthing environment can mean the difference between a harsh or gentle experience of birth. If it is long or difficult to move from bed to tub, if you must step up uncomfortably high to get into the tub, if you must support your own weight without something soft to sit or lean on, if there are machines humming or people rushing around to fill a tub that was not yet ready, if the water is too warm or too cool, you receive these as additional stresses and your one-pointed focus on yourself, your baby, and your process of birthing becomes diverted. The more you become diverted from your connection with your baby, the more the baby will begin to wonder what is happening and why you are being pulled away to handle something that frustrates your smooth flow rather than enhances it. These interruptions may seem minor and relatively easy to correct. However, from the hormone-heightened awareness of a birth, even a small obstacle seems large on your screen of perception.

Each person, object, or element becomes part of a whole, alive, emotionally and physically textured tapestry perceived from the center point of the MotherBaby unit. When you remember this view in preparing a birthing environment, the preparation becomes that of an artist's helper, laying out all the elements that you know will contribute to the artist creating a masterpiece. Birthing is art. The MotherBaby unit is the artist, and birth attendants are the artist's helpers. The point is not to control the environment in a static sense but to create an environment that moves with you and that you can easily move within. Often, women have thought they would deliver in a particular environment or a particular place within an environment and, to their surprise, ended up somewhere entirely different. One example is a woman thinking she would birth at home and ending up in a hospital or vice versa. For the birth of my son Hank, I thought I would birth outside in our hot tub and ended up birthing in the large bathtub adjacent to our bedroom.

When you and your baby are viewed as the central artists, environments, including birth attendants, must be flexible, for the attendants should not be demanding that you conform to their structure; they need to be willing to flow with you. The attendants become part of a birthing dance where all have come together in a mutual movement for the miracle of human life. You, as the mother, are also asked by the nature of things to trust the movement of your birth dance rather than some preconceived idea of how or where you thought you would be birthing. All must give in to what is authentically called forth. Sometimes, this might mean birthing in water when birthing in water was not planned, and sometimes the opposite. Something can authentically be called forth when all the elements that are desired are present and functional.

If you desire the element of water to be present in your birthing experience, it must not only be physically available but also available in the minds and spirits of those attending. This means that these people must feel confident and competent if water is used. Frequently, a woman has desired water in her birthing experience and had it physically available, but did not have attendants who felt confident or competent to support her in using it. Sometimes, the desire to use water is strong enough in the mother and possibly her partner that they use water in their delivery even though their attendants do not feel comfortable. Usually, however, the feeling that her attendants are uncomfortable outweighs her desire for using water, and a dry birth results, often with a feeling of disappointment that the option of water was not truly available for her.

The opposite can also occur when an attendant has such a strong desire for water to be used that the birthing mother feels she would be failing in what was expected of her if she did not use water in her birth. The main point in all this is that the creation of a birth experience involves a mutual giving in, or surrendering to, a deeper guiding force in that birthing experi-ence—a voice, if you will, that encompasses the greatest wisdom for all concerned. A birthing environment that acknowledges the presence of a deeper wisdom guiding the birthing experience will be an environment that miraculously has all the elements needed for the perfect artistic creation of a masterpiece in that birth.

The traffic flow in a birthing environment can be envisioned prior to the birth. What are the easiest pathways of movement to and from key locations (bathroom, bed, kitchen, supplies, tub, etc.) for the mother, family, and attendants? It is wise for you to ask your birth attendants to not only have a specific location in the space that is "home" for them when not needed to do some-thing else, but also to have a specific physical responsibility in the room, like keeping trash picked up, supplies organized, and being sure the midwife's or doctor's equipment is organized and not mixed with anything else. Often, birthing rooms, whether at home or in the hospital, will be fairly crowded with things and people, and it is important to be conscientious about the amount and direction of activity necessary while attending a birth. Remind your birth team that privacy is important to you (if it is) and that you will call them if you need them. If you are clear about such desires, birth team members will know to keep their activities, exams, talking, and observations to a minimum and to stay in the background, so your birthing energy is the central focus. It may be helpful to have an adjacent room where people can congregate or lie down and rest until you call them.

The quality of all the physical elements in a birthing environ-ment is also important. What is their shape, color, and texture? What kinds of feelings do they invoke? Do they function in the best way possible? What kind of lighting is available? If music is an element that is important to you and your family, is music easily available? What kind of music will contribute most to this birth masterpiece? If there is a desire to record the birth in some way, what method will be chosen, and can it be done in a way that is blended in with the natural flow of the birth itself?

Once the location—the "canvas" for the birth art—is selected, elements naturally begin to present themselves until the space feels complete. The location could be the hospital, home, birthing center, indoors, outdoors, bedroom, bathroom, living room, even the kitchen. Wherever you feel you will be the most comfortable and safe is usually the optimal place to plan for the birthing environment. Just remember that your plans may change in the moment. Michel Odent told me a story about a wealthy woman in London who planned a home birth with him. Since she was not sure in advance where she would want to birth, she had all the oriental rugs in her home covered in plastic, except under the grand piano, where she was sure she would not want to be. Yet, that was precisely the spot where she ended up giving birth because that turned out to be where she felt the safest and most protected.

I know a woman who selected seven things that were important to her to bring to her hospital birth: a large painting of a purple orchid which she hung on the hospital wall to gaze into during labor; a red silk shawl given to her by her mother; the music she had been listening to during her pregnancy, including ocean waves with dolphin sounds; a quilt that had been her grandmother's; two pillows from her own bed; and a vase of fresh flowers. This woman reported that the inclusion of these elements and the support of her husband and another friend made all the difference in the world in her feeling of comfort and assurance in her birth experience. Birthing environments can be as varied and infinite as there are birthing women and babies.

The birthing environment for my son Hank's birth was my large bathroom adjacent to the bedroom with a large oval bathtub. Above the tub was a stained-glass window, and in each corner of the tub were some fresh yellow and purple chrysanthemums. There were five candles burning in an otherwise dark room. My midwife and friends—including Robbie, whose birth story with me in attendance is in the preceding chapter—quietly entered the room and spontaneously and softly began to sing a chant we had sung at our birth meetings. The sound of their voices singing in quiet unity allowed me to go deeper within myself and be with Hank through each movement of his delivery. I relaxed my body so much when he came out that I felt ecstatic pleasure. The energy of the room felt like it had fabric to it, a warm vibrational receiving blanket for Hank.

SELECTION OF A TUB

Anything that holds water that is comfortable for the mother, that is non-toxic, easy to clean, fill, and drain would be appropriate for a water delivery. The tubs I have seen used most often are bathtubs, Jacuzzis, fiberglass hot tubs, galvanized steel tubs, and small inflatable pools. I also know of plastic kiddie swimming pools being used, a Japanese-made plastic hot tub, wooden hot tubs, a frame with a waterbed liner, a plexiglass tub, and quiet tidepools in the ocean. Home bathtubs, even the standard size, seem to work fine. I attended a birth in the Soviet Union that took place in a narrow bathroom tub. The mother squatted perpendicular to the length of the tub and birthed a beautiful little boy in about 20 inches of warm water. A benefit of home bathtubs is that they are already installed and easy to drain and fill. A drawback may be that they are usually open only on one side, and more difficult for attendants to be where they need to be to help. If the bathtub is small, it is not as easy for the father/partner to be in the tub with the mother for the delivery should the couple so desire. Another drawback to the standard-size bathtub is that you do not have as much freedom of movement in labor as you might like to have.

I felt secure birthing Hank in the familiarity of our own bathtub, which fortunately was quite large. You may also feel this way, especially if that tub is a place where you have spent some quiet moments during your pregnancy reflecting and being with your baby in utero. If you are planning to birth in a tub that is unfamiliar to you, I suggest you spend time in that tub days prior to the delivery to get accustomed to the tub by playing and relaxing in it, and visualizing receiving your baby.

Although not as aesthetically pleasing as some large bathtubs, galvanized steel tubs or inflatable tubs offer a portability and spaciousness that you may like (see Figures 3.1 and 3.2). Your tub can be placed a few steps from your bed, in an outdoor location, or some other special location, as long as it can be reached by a hose, usually connected to the hot water heater, and attached to an opening at the base of the tub. Through this hose water can be added or drained, although not as easily as in a regular bathtub. I used a 6-foot-long and 2-foot-wide steel tub in my daughter Mela's birth in 1980 and again in 1984 with my daughter Orien. As mine was, a steel tub can, for example, be painted in pastel shades of blue, pink, or green on the inside with a white exterior, perhaps with flowers on it. It seems that fathers or partners enjoy painting and preparing the tub for their baby's birth. It is an important ritual for the family to feel comfortable and connected with the tub that will be receiving the newest member of their family.

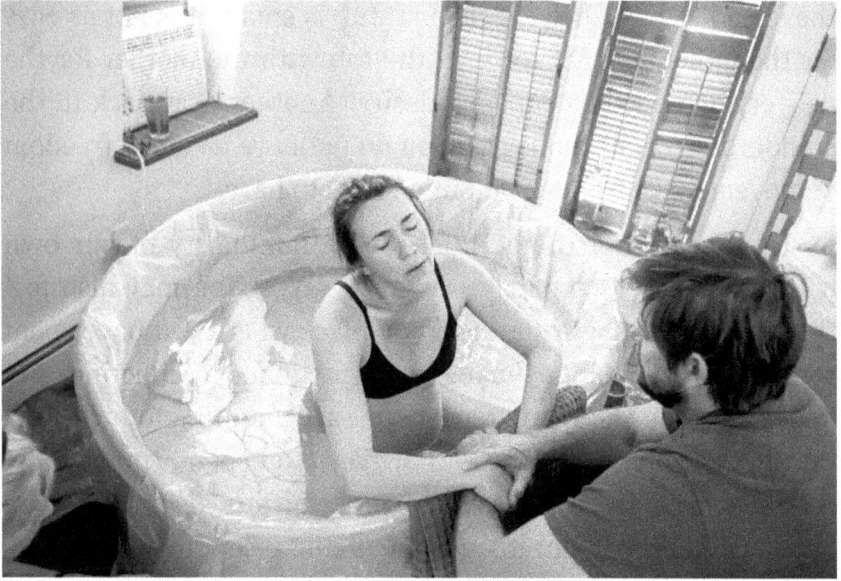

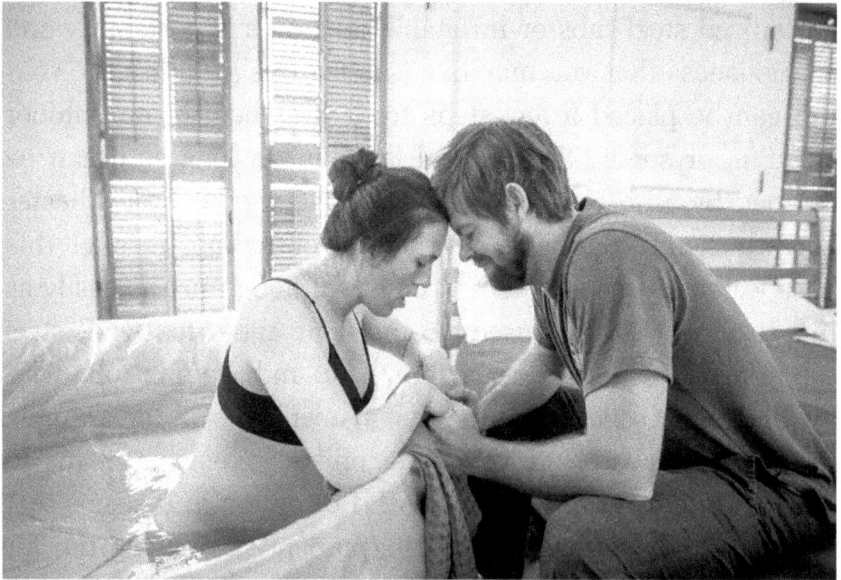

Figures 3.1 and 3.2. *My daughter Orien in "laborland" with her husband Andy in their inflatable tub, which they placed in their bedroom close to their bed and filled with a hose that they ran from a heater. Photo by Monet Nicole, used with permission.*

PREPARATION OF THE TUB AND THE WATER

Once the tub and its location are selected, it should be cleaned just prior to the birth. I used an iodine solution and filled the tub with only hot water, about halfway. This is especially necessary in homes where the hot water heater will need to reheat the water a couple of times until the tub will be full of warm water. The hot water can be sitting there cooling while you are in labor, and cold water to make the temperature just right can be added prior to you entering the tub. It is necessary to know how many gallons of water your tub holds and how long it will take to fill it with warm water. Often, mothers and babies are ready to get in before their tubs are ready. Michel Odent has noted that many mothers relax so much upon hearing the sound of running water that babies are born while the tub is being filled.

Beah Haber, a Certified Nurse-Midwife from Livermore, California, comments on the care of the tub used in her birth center:

> We have a four-person tub in our birth room which is supplied by a 200-gallon water heater ... After the birth we empty the tub and refill it with water and concentrated chlorine. The jets are turned on to let the chlorine circulate and we change the filter. The tub is emptied again and scrubbed with a strong disinfectant solution, and is given a final rinse with water. As a double-check, we run an environmental aerobic culture once a week if the tub was used.[1]

Ordinary tap water has been used in most water deliveries with no, or only rare, reporting of any infections in the mother. We used salt in the water in Mela's birth in 1980 because we were attempting to make the water as close to amniotic fluid as we could. It worked just fine, but later, we decided that plain tap water worked equally well. At that time, I learned that Michel Odent had used regular tap water in over 200 births in Pithiviers, France, with no incidence of infection. I have known people who have used distilled water in their tubs, others who have dechlorinated their water or prepared it in other special ways using homeopathic solutions, flower essences, or crystals. In addition to a clean tub and water, whatever ways feel good to you are the best ways to prepare the water for that particular birth. Comfortable water temperature seems to be between 95-101 degrees.

Other items helpful to have in a water delivery include foam sponges for the mother to kneel on if she so desires; a small birthing stool or something to sit on in the tub (I found this especially helpful after the delivery, when I wanted to sit upright in the tub to nurse my baby); inflatable bath pillows to lean against or float on; an aquarium net or some other kind of strainer to scoop vernix, feces, or other debris out of the water (this is a great job for a birth team member to feel useful); lots of towels, which are especially useful for birth team members to lean their elbows on; and cushions for birth attendants to kneel or sit on instead of a hard floor. Robbie has told me that in New Zealand, most tubs in birth centers and hospitals have vinyl cushions attached to their sides for this purpose (see Figure 3.3). You also can simply pull up a stool for your attendant to sit on next to the tub, as in Figure 3.4 below. If it is important to you to know the exact temperature of the water, a thermometer should be available.

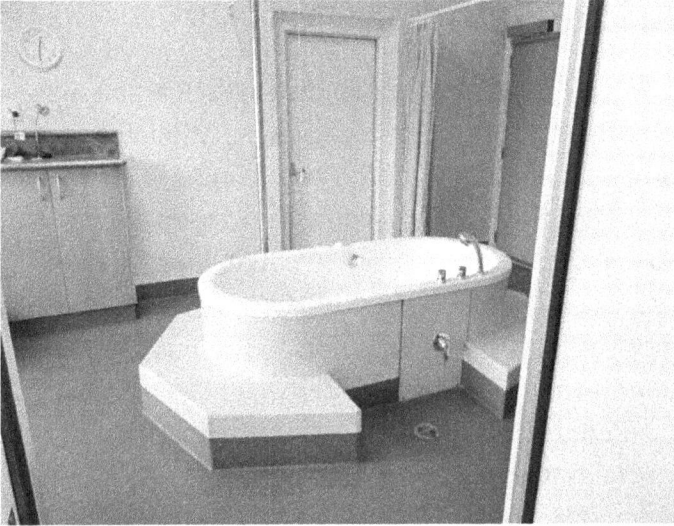

Figure 3.3. *A birthing tub in a New Zealand birth center with with a vinyl cushion for the midwives to sit or kneel on. Photo by Robbie Davis-Floyd, used with permission.*

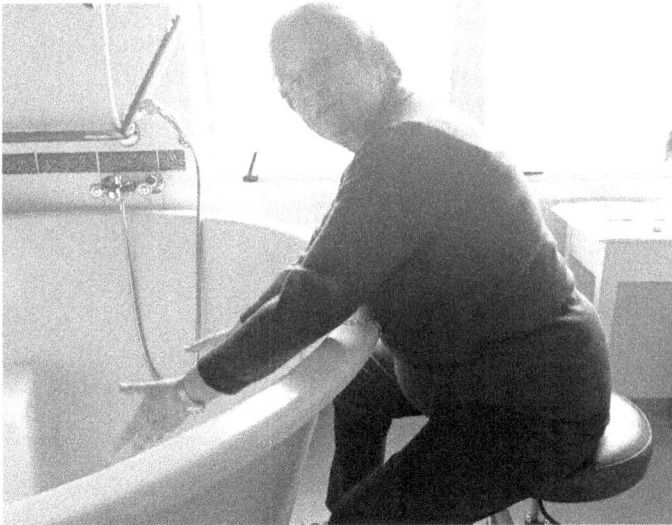

Figure 3.4. *Pulling up a mobile stool on wheels for the midwife to sit by the edge of the tub in another New Zealand birth center. Photo by Robbie Davis-Floyd, used with permission.*

THE BIRTH PROCESS IN WATER

If you are not already in the tub during labor, you may wish to wait to get in until you are 10 centimeters dilated and/or feeling the desire to push. Once in the tub, you will be able to move around and feel the positions you want to be in to help your body move the baby through the vaginal canal. Since your weight loss in water is equal to the weight of the water displaced, you can feel almost weightless because you are so buoyant in the water. I have found this feeling of greater weightlessness such a relief when I entered the tub during labor that I attribute it to my ability to relax and focus on the baby. My muscles simply did not have to work as hard to support or to move my body around. Psychologically, a warm bath is a cue for relaxing and letting go, and this certainly seems to hold true in birth.

Linda Church, a Certified Nurse-Midwife at the Family Birthing Center of Upland, California, comments on her experience of women who labor or birth in water: "She relaxes without using medication and experiences less pain. Her anxiety decreases, apparently reducing her adrenalin levels, thus encouraging her natural oxytocin and endorphins to flow uninhibited. A natural balance of pain and relaxation is achieved, and her labor progresses normally."[2]

Vital signs of temperature, pulse, or blood pressure can easily be taken when you are in a tub of water. Monitoring fetal heart tones can be done with a fetoscope if you move so that your belly is out of the water, or waterproof, wireless electronic fetal monitoring can be done if you are in a hospital that has this relatively new technology. A Doppler (which records the fetal heartbeat by use of sound waves) can be used underwater if sealed inside a plastic bag, so you do not have to leave the tub for your attendant to take the fetal heart tones (see Figure 3.5). Vital signs can be checked as often as you wish. If the father or other parent is planning to be in the tub to receive the baby, it is wise for that person to feel comfortable in warm water so they can stay in for a longer time than they may be used to. Often, the partner (or doula) holds the mother from behind so she can comfortably lean back and rest between contractions. This person becomes like a birthing chair for you.

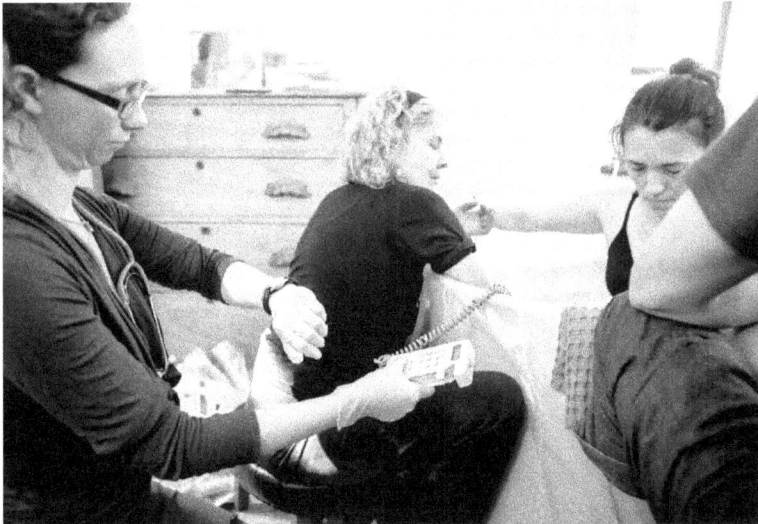

Figure 3.5. *Orien's two midwives check the fetal heart rate with a Doppler. Photo by Monet Nicole, used with permission.*

Delivery positions in warm water tend to be more flexible than on dry land and easier to maneuver according to the inner wisdom of the birthing flow. Sometimes, you may want to hang on someone so you can let your bottom and legs go, or you may want to squat and hold onto the sides of the tub. Other positions I have seen in tubs are hands and knees, semi-reclining, or lying on your side. Hands-and-knees or "all-fours" positions are particularly beneficial, as they allow for maximal pelvic opening.[3] Yet, any position that feels good to you, and in which you can totally let go, is the best position for that delivery. Dry births in upright or all-fours positions have the benefit of gravity to help the mother deliver. In dry births, attendants may use warm water packs or warm oil to massage and help stretch the perineum. Being immersed in warm water has the same effect of relaxing and helping the perineum to stretch, most of the time without the need for any additional perineal support.

The Number One question people ask when they hear of babies being delivered in water is, "Why doesn't the baby drown?" I have heard Michel Odent answer that question: "Babies are very intelligent. They know not to breathe underwater." Odent and others have observed that it is the contact with the atmosphere that stimulates a baby to breathe and not just that the baby comes out of the womb (see Figures 3.6 and 3.7).

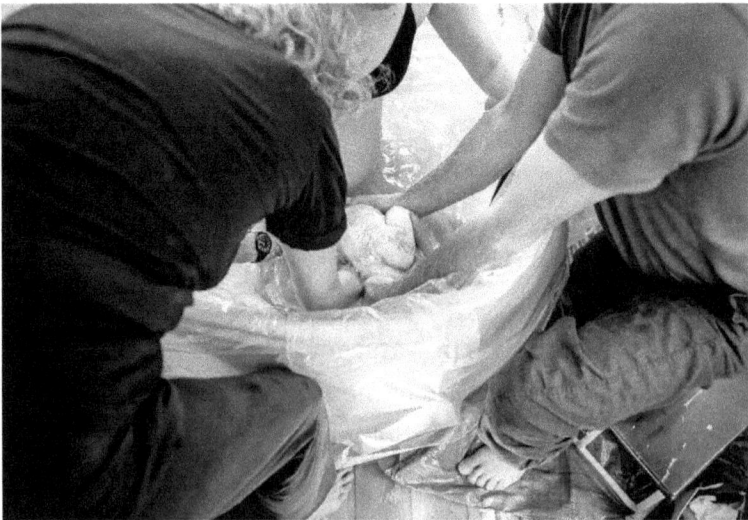

Figure 3.6. *My daughter Orien giving birth to my grandson Eli in the water. The cord had been wrapped around his neck. Here, you see the midwife gently removing it. Photo by Monet Nicole, used with permission.*

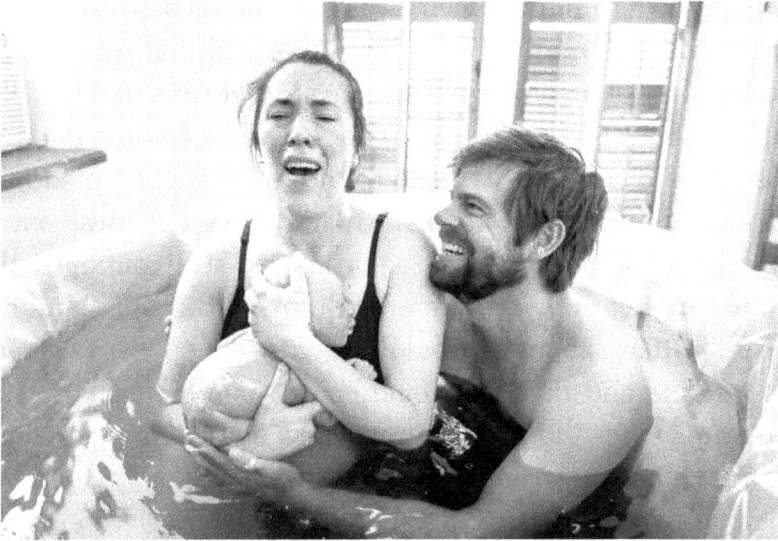

Figure 3.7. *Newborn ecstasy! Photo by Monet Nicole, used with permission.*

Dr. John Bastyr, founder of the college of naturopathic medicine in Seattle, Washington, attended many water deliveries in the 1930s and 1940s. He had been advising his pregnant clients to labor in a warm bath to ease pain, and there came a time when a woman would not get out of the tub for the delivery. Dr. Bastyr said he had about nine seconds to decide if a baby would drown if it came out underwater: "I reasoned the baby had been in water for nine months, the placenta and umbilical cord would still be attached and functioning after the baby came out, babies do not drown in the womb, so they would not drown in the extended womb of a warm bath." He said his decision that water delivery was perfectly fine and the baby's actual delivery were just about simultaneous: "I gently lifted the baby out of the water into his mother's arms and all were very happy. After that birth, I found that more and more women did not want to leave the bath for their delivery!"[4]

In my own thinking, when I was considering delivering Mela, my first daughter, in warm water, I reasoned that warm water had been my baby's natural environment for nine months, and what would feel more strange to her would be coming into dryness and direct gravity. I thought the warm water would be a gift for her, an acknowledgment that although she was out of her original womb, her new environment still contained the familiar element of warm water with my body still around her. I also felt that she and I would have just done lots of work in birthing her and that she would enjoy some moments to rest in a familiar medium to integrate the work she had just done. She could then move on to the next new stimuli of direct sound, touch, air, and gravity. It is a marvel to me how nature allows for this integration time, whether on land or in water, through having a placenta and umbilical cord that remain functioning and supplying oxygen to the baby for up to ten minutes or more after delivery. I and many others find it disconcerting that in the hospital, the umbilical cord is often cut immediately after delivery, thereby cutting babies off from their oxygen supply just as they are trying to take their first breaths of air. The umbilical cord should not be cut until it stops pulsing, for as long as it is pulsing, the baby is still receiving oxygenated blood from the placenta.

Often during delivery, the baby's head will be out some moments before the body is delivered. Once born, the baby may rest underwater for a few moments. This can be a tense or an ecstatic moment, depending on the perceptions of the people viewing it. It is true that a few babies born into water have drowned because their midwife or parent kept them under the water for too long, usually for ideological reasons: some people, especially in Russia, who were under the influence of Dr. Igor Charkovsky—whom I discuss later in this chapter—used to believe that human babies were like dolphin babies and could immediately adapt to the water environment, and so should stay in it for quite a while after delivery.[5] Few people now hold this belief. Drowning is easy to avoid—simply draw your baby up to you soon after delivery, or allow the newborn to swim to the surface if that is what they decide to do. It is important for you and your midwives, doctors, or other birth facilitators to have their own experience of knowing and feeling that it is safe for the baby to come out in water. We may know in our conscious minds that many thousands of babies have been delivered in water and are perfectly healthy and alive, but we need to also know in our hearts and our emotions that water delivery is just as safe as land delivery. (Anywhere in the world, even in the wealthiest hospitals in the highest-resource countries, out of every 1000 land births, at least 2 babies will die. That rate does not rise with home delivery nor with water delivery.[6]) Until birth attendants have this experience of "knowingness" integrated in their being, I recommend that they not be the person primarily responsible for a water delivery. It does not have to be a long process to come to this "knowingness" about water delivery, as Dr. Bastyr has shown us, but it may.

The five randomized controlled trials on waterbirth conducted to date have shown that benefits for mothers include lower pain scores, less use of pain medication, less use of artificial oxytocin, shorter labors, a higher rate of normal vaginal birth, a higher rate of intact perineums, less use of episiotomy, and greater satisfaction with the birth. Another study found that fewer people in the waterbirth group had cesareans compared to people in the land birth group (5% versus 16%). There was less meconium (the baby's first stool) in the mother's amniotic fluid with waterbirth (2% versus 24%), and fewer low Apgar scores with waterbirth compared to land birth. (An Apgar score is a test of how well the baby is doing at birth. A low Apgar score means that the baby may require medical assistance.) No babies have died in the water in any of the many studies conducted.[7]

Yet, even after a person has the statistics on the safety of water birth, they may need additional time to do the inner work it may take to believe it and feel it. Birth attendants are valuable people, and it is important for them to be present with birthing families from their own authentic experience, not just from what they think they should or should not be doing in their birth practices.

Beah Haber, certified nurse-midwife, talks about her transition to deeply knowing the safety of water births:

> When I first heard about women having their babies in water, I reacted by reciting all of the arguments which have now become too familiar: "If we were meant to give birth in water, we'd have gills ... How do you know when that baby will take its first breath? ... It doesn't seem natural ..." A few years later, I attended a woman who labored in water and refused to give in to our gentle prodding to get out of the water for the actual birth. As I watched, I was surprised by several things. Inside me, I found trust of the process instead of fear, a feeling that had initially drawn me to birth itself. I didn't find myself holding my breath until the baby first took hers, but instead joined the mother and her baby in a very quiet, restful focus.[8]

Virginia Jackson, Maria Corsaro, and Cynthia Niles, certified nurse-midwives in New York, comment on how they reacted to women who did not want to leave their labor bath for delivery: "Our lack of experience with, and suspicion of, underwater birth led us to thwart these women's instincts, urges, and desires ... It is our clients who have shown us the benefits of water for comfort in labor and who have guided us to comfort with underwater birth."[9]

To see a baby's head and face emerge from another human being's body, whether immersed in air or water, can be a life-transforming event. It is difficult for most people to believe that what they are seeing is happening, for it is so miraculous that one whole human being, whom they have never seen before, is coming from within another whole human being. Even when we think we understand how such an event came about through sperm, egg, chromosomes, and cell division, when confronted by the actual emergence of the baby's head at delivery, through a process that, despite all our efforts, remains relatively uncontrollable, we are amazed. Transfixed, we seem to be viewing the impossible becoming possible before our very eyes. About watching my daughter Orien being born into water, my friend Robbie said, "It was as if she were emerging from a star-studded distant galaxy, far, far away, or coming from another dimension into ours."

Physicians and midwives who have witnessed thousands of deliveries have told me that they are continually touched by the miracle of each one. Michel Odent has said, "Being present at the birth of thousands of babies changes you into a different person—as long as the births are not too disturbed by the medical establishment. The holy atmosphere of a birthing room is catching. And to share this holy atmosphere gives you a more global vision. It helps you sort out the essential from matters of secondary importance."[10]

In birth, we are witnessing something that was totally invisible to us previously now becoming visible. Each person must confront the question, "Where did this baby come from?" To ask and answer this question, for most people, involves looking at their relationship with the "holy." As Michel Odent has noted, this experience of being in the presence of the holy is a daily experience for those who witness birth and are open to experiencing its sacredness and holiness. "Holy" comes from the root word for "whole," and the root word for whole is "health." The nature of viewing a birth is to ask us to see wholeness. We are asked to actually see the visible and invisible being one. We are asked to see the wholeness of the mother begetting the wholeness of the baby. We are asked to see the wholeness of the male and female merging to create life. We are asked to see our eyes looking back at us through this new baby's eyes. All around us, at birth, we are asked to see the unity of all things. Even when we could say that a particular birth was fraught with much disunity, at the delivery of a whole child, we are faced with unity once again. Even disunity and unity join together in wholeness, in health. We are asked to face the incomprehensible "is-ness" of life. Although hospital practitioners may experience it as such, birth is *never* a mundane event (see Figures 3.8 and 3.9).

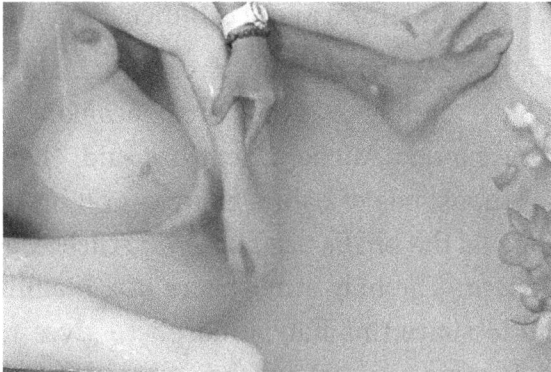

Figure 3.8. *A water birth in Bali at Bumi Sehat, a world-famous birthing center founded and operated by the 2011 CNN Hero of the Year, midwife Ibu Robin Lim, CPM. She created a tradition of scattering flowers in the water. Not only do they add color, but also a sense of sacredness, as flower petals are also used to make offerings to ancestor spirits. Photo by Robbie Davis-Floyd, used with the permission of the laboring woman.*

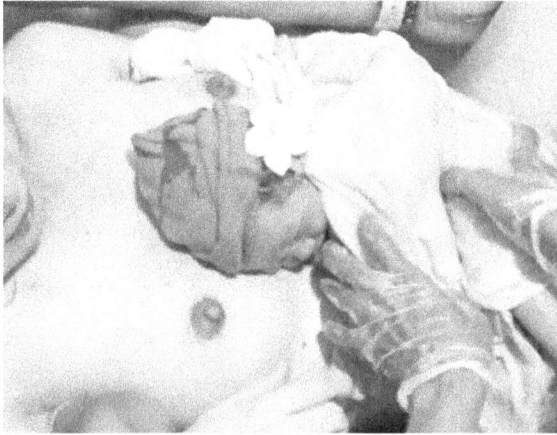

Figure 3.9. *The baby, too, is adorned with a flower. Photo by Robbie Davis-Floyd, used with the couple's permission.*

In birth, we may look at our relationship with wholeness. If in our own primal experiences, we are bonded to separation outside the context of wholeness, and the seeming necessity for separation in order to survive, then when we face the holiness (wholeness) of the baby, those separation/survival beliefs become activated. We feel we must do something to segment the wholeness in some way so that we can feel sure of survival. Once we feel in control through intervening in and segmenting the experience, we feel safe. However, the very nature of wholeness is the nature of being out of control. If something is whole, what is there that needs to be brought under control? All that needs to be there, including control, is there within the whole. It just is.

Human beings tend to want to take an experience that feels out of their control (and when surrendered to, usually feels pleasurable) and control it in some way, even if it is only through understanding this un-understandable event that just happened to them. We just are this way. We tend to resist the "peace that passeth all understanding" (see Figure 3.10).

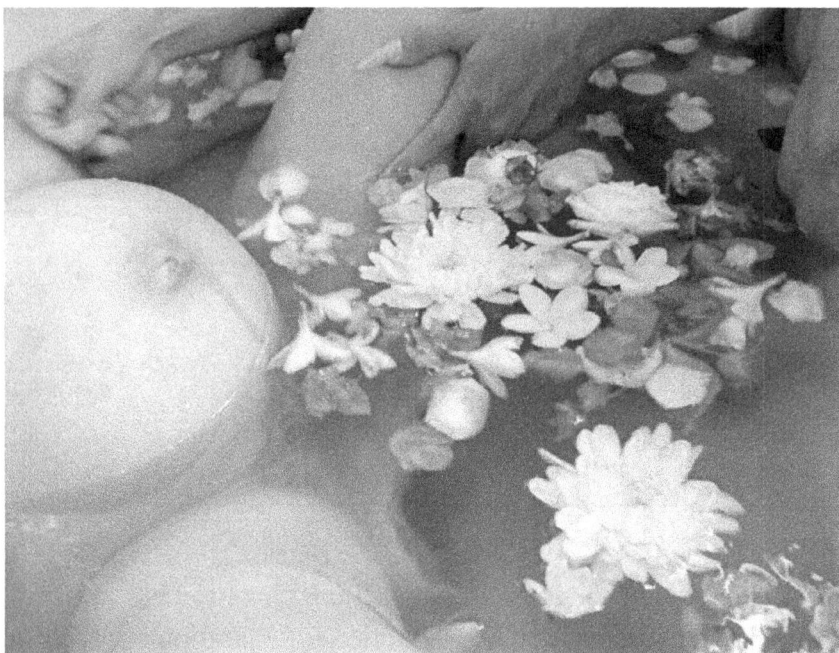

Figure 3.10. *A peaceful, sacred Balinese birth at Bumi Sehat, filled with beauty. Photo by Robbie Davis-Floyd, used with permission.*

In birth, as in life, when we deny that the part and the whole are one, we move into fear and the need for control. To see a baby emerge in the water and to be in denial that the medium of water is an appropriate place for entry into this world is to most definitely introduce fear and the desire to control into the birthing experience. When we remember that most of our planet is water, it seems ludicrous to deny human babies the right to emerge in that medium if they so desire. Perhaps they are attempting to bridge some kind of gap between land and water to show us that these elements are not mutually exclusive to one another. It is my strong opinion that mothers and babies deserve to be as wet or as dry as they want to be in birth.

To consider that babies grow and develop in the medium of water within their mother's womb is to add more rationality to their choice to connect with water outside the womb. Maybe we just do not need, as much as we once did in the evolutionary cycle, to deny and separate ourselves from the environment from which we originated. Maybe this third choice (other than stay or go, here or there) to become all that we have been in an interwoven continuum of harmony is becoming more plausible. When people who attend births are able to hold this view as possible, they may come to perceive births in water as just as normal as births in air. Then, when a birth attendant sees a baby emerge in water, they see just as much wholeness, unhampered by fear or control, as they see when babies emerge in air.

This same hypothesis about denial, fear, and control can be applied to home and hospital births. If a birth attendant is in denial that the home is an appropriate place to give birth, they-would be in fear and control in that setting and unable to see the possibility for wholeness there. The same is true in reverse. If a birth attendant is in denial that the hospital is an appropriate place to give birth, they would be in fear and control in that setting and unable to perceive wholeness. *When we deny any aspect of reality and see it as disconnected from us, we will be in fear and will want to control that aspect rather than reconnect with it.* It is wonderful to have ideas, opinions, and preferences about birth. We serve people when we express the insights and meaning birth has for us. However, when these preferences become demands or rules about the right way to birth, we deny the infinite variety of realities that are possible in birth on Earth.

In water deliveries, when babies emerge into the air, they may spit fluids out of their mouths or make swallowing motions. Intrauterine photography has shown us that babies swallow and spit out amniotic fluids while in the womb. These motions are normal as long as the heart tones are fine and there is plenty of oxygen through the umbilical cord. It is interesting to note the intensity with which some practitioners still ensure that babies have fluids suctioned out of their noses, mouths, and throats immediately after birth; such suctioning is not actually needed. When you think that this creature has been living perfectly well for nine months in water and has been given the gift of a transition period with the umbilical cord still pulsing as in the womb, you begin to wonder just whose benefit such instantaneous suctioning is really for, and to realize that it's really for the benefit of practitioners.

When your baby emerges in the water, it is important that the heart tones be checked, as well as the pressure in the umbilical cord, and to watch for signs of the placenta separating from the uterine wall. As long as the heart tones are normal, over 100 beats per minute, cord pressure is strong, and you are not having strong uterine contractions, you can wait for you and the baby to mutually decide when to bring the baby to the surface for air-breathing. I find that mothers and babies usually know the perfect time to come to the surface to learn to breathe and to be brought to the breast. Most often, this amount of time seems to be from a few seconds up to two minutes. My daughter Mela (1980) was underwater for six minutes, Orien (1984) for 20 seconds, and Hank (1987) for one minute.

While underwater, your baby may open his eyes and look at you, your partner, and the other people present. He may move his arms and legs in stretching motions, or he may rest in a sleep-like state. Often babies smile, and sometimes they grimace and release stresses from coming through the birth canal. Carla Strange, certified nurse-midwife, speaks about a water delivery she attended: "As the baby emerged, I felt the pulsations of the cord, and we watched intently as she stretched her arms and grimaced her face. Her eyes were wide open, and she made a 'coughing' movement to spurt mucus from her mouth."[11] Another midwife, Beah Haber, comments: "As the baby was born, she opened her eyes and focused on one person after another around her. Her gaze was clear and thoughtful."[12] Mela smiled at us while underwater and sought eye contact with each of the people in the room.

I do not feel it is better for a baby to be left underwater for a longer amount of time or that there is one length of time that is right for all babies. I do feel that babies should not be rushed to the surface unless there is a medical reason to do so, or that is what the mother intuitively feels is correct. Most of us, at our births, were rushed to learn to breathe by premature cutting of the umbilical cord, so breathing was not a pleasurable thing but a matter of survival. This subconscious memory may cause you to want to rush your baby to breathe at birth. If, however, your baby has plenty of oxygen from the umbilical cord, there is no reason to rush. Relax, be in the moment, and take this next step in your birth dance together.

As previously mentioned, Apgar scoring is a method of evaluating and recording in numbers the condition of the baby at one minute and five minutes after birth.[13] Five vital signs of color, respiration, heartbeat, muscle tone, and response to flicking the foot are each given a score of 0-2 points. Ordinarily, a baby who receives a 2 for each point, resulting in an overall Apgar score of 10, would be completely pink, with a strong cry, heartbeat over 100 beats per minute, active movement of limbs, not limp, and cries in response to flicking the foot. In water deliveries, crying as a positive response is sometimes replaced by alertness and the obvious conscious presence of the baby. Virginia Jackson states: "The infants are usually in a relaxed pose; but their hands clench and unclench, indicating tone. The baby has an alert expression but usually does not cry."[14] The Family Birthing Center reports on 483 water deliveries; "The Apgar scores for all water births range from 6-9 at one minute, and 8-10 at five minutes."[15]

When bringing the baby up to begin air-breathing, some parents lay the baby in a safety position in their arms – face down with the head slightly downward so if there are any fluids to drain out, they will do so easily. Again, there is no need to routinely suction newborn babies, whether born in water or on land.

Most mothers hold their babies in their arms next to the left breast, which is close to the heartbeat, while they learn to breathe. Usually, all that is out of the water is the baby's face so that the rest of the body is still submerged. The baby may breathe right away or take his or her time. The cord is still intact, and there is no hurry as long as the baby is conscious, present, and connecting in his or her own way. Many parents talk or sing to their baby, welcoming him/her into the world. After we lifted her out of the water, Mela began breathing in tiny, almost imperceptible breaths for about the first minute. Then, she took a deep breath, and I could hear her lungs open up. She did not cry but looked attentive and alert. Carla Strange had a similar experience in a birth she attended: "This baby's first breath was quiet ... I was amazed at her presence and calm. Her breath was so still that I got my stethoscope and listened to her lungs for my own satisfaction, finding them perfectly clear. It was a beautiful birth."[16] When Orien was born, she came out of the water, took a big breath right away, and was ready to suckle. Hank took about a minute to gradually open up his breath and was also desirous of eye-to-eye contact.

This time in the tub after the delivery of the baby but before the delivery of the placenta is a special time for bonding between you and your baby. Often, the dad or partner enjoys holding the baby and floating the baby gently through the water. It is easy to see the baby's enjoyment and happiness in the water while, at the same time, being able to connect eye-to-eye with you. Such a welcome surprise of love for all! Jackson, Corsaro, and Niles comment: "The tub was large enough for her and her new son to spend several minutes relaxing in the water (the baby's head was out of the water). It was wonderful to view firsthand just how much this newborn enjoyed the water. His body was relaxed, his face alert and responsive. His mother was enthralled with the ease of her birth and the beauty of her baby."[17]

BIRTH COMPLICATIONS

Webster's Dictionary defines "complicate" as: "To combine especially in an involved or inextricable manner; to make complex or difficult." "Complex" comes from the Latin "to embrace, to comprise a multitude of objects." "Complication" is defined as "a difficult factor or issue often appearing unexpectedly and changing existing plans, methods, or attitudes; a secondary condition developing in the course of a primary condition."

Each birth experience is unique. Each has its own timing, character, and nuances. When a birthing process occurs in a normal, physiological way, with only a certain amount of information and stress to be handled by you, your baby, and your attendants, none of which is life-threatening, birth is said to be "uncomplicated." When a birthing becomes more complex or intricate, with an increase of information and stress that needs to be handled by you, your baby, and your attendants, and may be seen as life-threatening to you or your baby, a birth is said to be "complicated."

It is unique in the birthing process that women so often are also brought to look at death or the threat of death. It is as if what was "dead" (gone, unseen) to us is coming into life through birth, and this is such an awesome occurrence that we care intensely that this new being be born alive. It seems such a waste to the ego-mind for a being to die at birth, and given our own relationship to the transition of death, we can develop an inordinate demand that the outcome of all births be a live, healthy baby. "Life at any cost" can be seen as a summary of an extreme and rigid commitment to aliveness at birth.

As birth professionals know, and as we know from the deaths attributed to sudden infant death syndrome (SIDS), there is no way to absolutely guarantee the absence of mortality in birth. No matter what ingenious ways we come up with to assure the birth of live babies, death still seems to manage to occur. The perinatal mortality rate is defined by WHO as the number of stillbirths and deaths in the first week of life per 1,000 total births. The perinatal period commences at 28 weeks of gestation and ends 7 days after birth. As I mentioned above, no matter where we give birth nor how we deal with it, around 2 out of every 1000 babies will die at birth or shortly after. That is the ideal perinatal mortality rate, and it is achieved in midwife-attended home and freestanding birth center births in the U.S., in part because those births are low-risk and in part due to midwives' many skills[18], but not in hospital births, because hospitals attend to high-risk births as well. The perinatal mortality rate for the United States was 6/1000 in 2016, according to the latest data available. This rate ranged by state from a low of 4.33 in Wyoming to a high of 8.32 in Alabama and Mississippi. Black babies die or are born prematurely at higher rates than others. This appears to be due to the constant stress Black women experience from the systemic racism that still prevails in the U.S.[19] In any case, the fact remains that deaths occur at birth, both maternal and fetal, no matter what precautions or interventions have been attempted.

If you approach birth with a holistic viewpoint, you embrace the possibility of death at birth, not from a consciousness of fear and hatred of death but from a consciousness of wholeness. No matter what you believe about what happens between death and birth or between birth and death, the fact that births and deaths occur is obvious. Wholeness calls upon you to accept both possibilities within the unconditionality of your heart, without a demand for either one to occur. To admit to the real possibility that babies die at birth and that you may birth a baby who dies is terrifying. It can, indeed, be alarming to know that you cannot control the outcome of a birth, no matter how much you might like to. To know this and yet to proceed as a parent, midwife, nurse, doctor, or birth facilitator is remarkable. It is also mandatory, in my opinion.

If you refuse to unconditionally accept the risk of death in childbirth, you will be basing your actions on the need to avoid death by attempting to control that possibility out of existence. This stance is in large part responsible for the malpractice crisis in obstetrics. No one wants to be responsible for death or near-death in birth. Since we have not yet been able to totally control this possibility, it behooves us to accept it and move on from that vantage point. Doing so can give everyone more freedom in the birthing experience, for your actions will not be coming from fear but from a deeper sense of what is right or purposeful in each unique situation. Certainly, you desire for you and your baby to be alive, healthy, and happy at birth! Giving up your resistance to the possibility of death magically gives you a greater chance to manifest your original desire.

It has been my experience that the underlying cause of most complications in birth is fear: fear of death, fear of being out of control, fear that you will have to trust something from beyond what you know with your ego-mind. These fears in birth are often caused by unconscious patterns, usually from your own birth experiences and/or from family patterns related to birth. If these patterns are not examined beforehand, they tend to become visible in some way during birth. For example, long labors, breech presentations, cesarean births, and other distinct patterns tend to follow family lines. If your mother had an induced birth with drugs, you may tend to recreate a similar birth for your children. If you were birthed in a relatively normal and easy way by your mother, you may tend to have normal, easy births with your children. In water birth, as in all births, it is important to obtain a family history of birth from the mother, father, and anyone else who is significantly involved.

Birth attendants also attract complications in their practices that reflect their own birth patterns. Dr. Graham Farrant, an Australian psychiatrist, told me of an obstetrician he worked with who found he "had" to use forceps in almost all of his deliveries. In his therapy sessions with Dr. Farrant, this obstetrician remembered and reexperienced his own birth with forceps. After this experience, this obstetrician found he no longer had to use forceps in most of his deliveries. He simply had been unable to see any differently due to his own unhealed birth experience. I have also known some birth attendants who have had unusually high numbers of breech deliveries and who themselves were delivered breech. (Breech deliveries account for only around 3% of all births worldwide.)

I was born by cesarean section. The doctor who performed the cesarean on my mother was also my doctor for the birth of my first child, a son who later accidentally died at age 4. I was twenty years old and not particularly prepared for any type of birth, nor did I have any conscious understanding of family patterns in birth. I simply did what I was told in the midst of tremendous fear that I would die giving birth. The birth took twenty-four hours, and my son was delivered with forceps. Hours after the birth, my physician told me that if he had known how small my pelvis was, he would have done a cesarean. "I'm sure any other births you have will have to be cesarean," he said. Upon hearing him, I remember feeling a great deal of relief and thought: "He is right. That would be the right way for me to have a baby." In having that thought, I was following my own family pattern.

For Mela's birth twelve years later, in order to break that pattern, I prepared myself with much information and knowledge for a normal vaginal delivery. I had reexperienced much of my own birth and felt much safer with the whole birth process. Yet during labor with Mela, I still had thoughts and feelings that said, "Can my body really birth this baby vaginally?" I asked my attendants to verbally support me by telling me I was doing the right thing and that my body was perfectly suited to give birth vaginally. This supported me in what I knew to be the real truth for me and allowed me to relax and release any fears and doubts I still had.

Many of the modern interventions of obstetrics do help mothers and babies in some cases. However, it has been proven that they also give rise to more interventions, which complicate the birth process further and result in less desirable outcomes for the mother and baby. A major example in the United States is the use of the favored lithotomy position for delivery. In this position, the birthing woman is lying flat on a table with feet in stirrups. This position compresses the pelvic outlet, making it much harder for the mother to push the baby through. The mother and baby are actually having to push uphill against gravity to deliver, and the large blood vessel sending oxygenated blood to the baby is depressed, often causing distress (erratic or lowered heartbeat) in the infant. When this occurs, a doctor may feel justified to intervene further to "help" the baby get out by doing an episiotomy (cutting the mother's perineum) and pulling the baby out with forceps or a vacuum extractor. This suction cup is fitted over the baby's head to pull the baby out. Nancy Wainer Cohen and Lois Estner, authors of *Silent Knife: Cesarean Prevention and Vaginal Birth after Cesarean*, ask:

> Is the slowly progressing woman walking and taking nourishment and squatting when she pushes? Is she offered kind words and gentle encouragement when she becomes dehydrated? Or is she lying flat on her back, I.V. in place, fetal monitor clattering away, food and drink denied, and all manner of analgesia and anesthesia offered when she shows signs of frustration?[20]

When these interventions are used because of fear and distrust of the natural process of birth, they actually manifest the nightmares they were supposedly created to avoid.[21] When such interventions are used only in the service of the natural process of birth, they can be helpful, and the number of times they are needed would be drastically reduced.

A case in point is the cesarean epidemic in the United States. Currently, one out of three women will have a cesarean section, and many of these women will accept it as a commonplace event. Yet, as recently as 1970, the overall cesarean birth rate in the U.S. was 6%, a rate deemed normal by generations of obstetric and nursing textbooks.[22] But after the electronic fetal monitor was introduced in that same year, over the next ten years, the cesarean rate rose to 23%, largely because the monitor registers every fetal heart rate drop—most of which are normal—often leading practitioners to think the baby is in distress when it is not.[23] I note again that, according to the World Health Organization, the cesarean birth rate should be no higher than 10%-15%. Yet, in the U.S., it has stood at around 32% for the past ten years and is much higher in many other countries, in what is called the "global cesarean epidemic."

The use of cesarean sections has been an attempt to avoid risk in birth. A doctor in one of my lectures told me he felt confident that the baby and mother would be alive if he did a cesarean, but he did not have the same confidence if the birth was allowed to take its own course. He also told me he did not think it was such a bad idea for all births to be by cesarean section. When one views the human body as a machine, it is easier to see from the doctor's viewpoint. The birth becomes simply a mechanical procedure that should be done in the most expedient way possible. This doctor went on further to tell me that he thought women would be grateful not to have to go through the pain of labor. Overall, he felt—and he is not alone—that the rapid rise in cesarean sections was a positive sign for birth in the United States. Yet Cohen and Estner ask, "Why did we relinquish our rights as healthy, normal birthing women and join the ranks of ailing hospital patients? When did we start believing that surgical delivery is safer and better for our babies?"[24]

Michel Odent has often said, "The first aim of obstetrics is always to control the delivery, while our aim [at the hospital in Pithiviers, France] is not to control the delivery but to support the birthing woman to be instinctual."[25] What we see in this controversy between controlled and non-controlled birth is a split in consciousness. One side totally fears nature, and the other totally fears technology. It also appears, coincidentally, that as consumer demand for natural birth rose, the cesarean section rate also rose. Robbie Davis-Floyd addressed this issue:

> Over 70% of all American obstetricians have been sued ... Malpractice insurance premiums in obstetrics began their dramatic rise in 1973, just when the natural childbirth movement was beginning to pose a major threat to the obstetrical paradigm ... Consequently, the explosion of humanistic and holistic options that challenge the conceptual hegemony of the technological model has been paralleled by a stepping up of ritual performance, in the form of a dramatic rise in the use of the fetal monitor (from initial marketing in the 1970s to near-universal hospital use today), accompanied by a concurrent rise in the cesarean rate.[26]

Robbie identifies "science, technology, patriarchy, and institutions" as core values of U.S. society, and sees the interests of these as superseding the interests of "nature, families, individuals, and women." When these are seen in opposition to each other, problems will result, for each side will be denying themselves the benefits of the other.[27] Obstetricians, in electing cesareans over natural birth, will be denying themselves the benefit of witnessing the power, strength, and flexibility of a mother and baby as they move through the mysterious, ancient miracle of birth. Do-it-yourself homebirth advocates will be denying themselves the potential benefits of the wisdom and support of modern technology. Both sides of this split in consciousness must be able to see the value in each side and embrace one another, rather than cling to rightness and separation.

Most of us have been raised and bonded to the technological model of reality—or what Robbie now calls "the technocratic model of reality"[28]—as it has been the dominant force in our culture for over fifty years. In order to see the benefits in the nature side of the split, we have had to, sometimes radically, alter our perceptions. Robbie speaks of this change in consciousness:

> To shift to the other side of the paradigm is to question and ultimately reject the ideas that the body is a machine and the mind somehow separate from it, that the institution is the most important social unit, that science and technology should attempt to dominate and control nature, that patriarchy is better than equality. It is to uphold the family as the most significant social unit (hence the holistic inclusion of the father/partner and siblings at births). It is to place science and technology at the service of the individual. It is to honor and celebrate women and men as equal and complementary partners in their search for individual growth and cultural evolution, and to honor the Earth as a living being engaged in her own evolutionary quest—a process in which our science and technology must become her allies instead of her enemies. It is a shift of such significance that it has the potential to transform American society.[29]

When you look at the potential for complications in birth, you must also look at consciousness, which includes beliefs, thoughts, feelings, and physiology. It is my theory that the more you identify with one side of the paradigm in separation from the other side, the more likely you will be to have a complicated birth. Instead of fighting one another, hospital birthers and home birthers, obstetricians and midwives, should support one another. Hospital birthing rooms should become more like home, and home birthing rooms should become more like the hospital – in other words, midwives who practice home birth should be proficient in the use of certain supportive technologies (as almost all of them are), and doctors who practice non-interventive, caring, natural birth in the hospital should not be laughed out of town for "pandering" to the demands of women and thereby being "irresponsible."

Leo Sorger, natural birth obstetrician, has said, "More and more frequently today, we doctors are being asked to stop hiding behind our scientific tools and to practice our art."[30] It is truly when the art and science of birth merge that we will have the most wholesome, natural, safe, and joyous birth experiences for our families.

Water and Pain in Labor and Delivery

Using warm water to ease the pain of powerful contractions in labor and delivery is well understood by women who have experienced it. In my first delivery in a hospital setting, I received painkillers to help ease my labor. I remember swearing to the nurse that she was giving me nothing. I could feel no difference. Years later, when I felt such intensity in Mela's birth that I did not know how I would go on, I entered a warm bath. The experience was one of such immediate relief and relaxation that I dilated two centimeters almost immediately. My experience is not unique. In speaking of his observations at Pithiviers, Michel Odent states:

> The woman immerses herself in warm water, often up to her neck. Sometimes an attentive hand gently supports her head while her ears are submerged. In the pool, labor becomes easier, more comfortable, less painful, and more efficient ... We tend to reserve our pools for women who have painful and inefficient contractions at around five centimeters' dilation. But water can be relaxing for the others, too. It can be as comforting as a lover, a mother, or a midwife.[31]

Water, by its very nature, is fluid, flexible, flowing—the very qualities a birthing woman needs to open up and release her baby. Michel Odent comments on women who told him they did not like water or could not swim: "Yet as labor begins, these same women will suddenly move toward the pool, enter eagerly, and not want to leave!"[32] These women seemed to know, in birthing their babies, that the water was there like a friend to help them rather than something to be feared, as they had previously thought.

Using warm water to ease pain in labor and delivery is probably the most often cited reason women give for their choice to use water in their birthing experience. One woman I interviewed said, "Warm water helped me to feel comfortable, and when I felt comfortable, I relaxed, even though the power of the contractions was the same. When I relaxed, the pain I was feeling disappeared, and I felt incredible energy moving through me, but it was not 'pain' as I had experienced it before."

Leboyer has said that "pain is resistance" and, again, as many therapists say, "What you resist, persists." If water, which is not resistant to anything, can be the stimulus to help a birthing woman give up her resistance to powerful contractions, what a simple "miracle" we have to assist birthing women. There is no need to hook her up to anything, to give her drugs that may or may not be harmful to her and her baby, or to watch her suffer through contractions in the midst of resistance. The element of water, which makes up 75 percent of our bodies and our planet, so naturally lends its support to the *superfluid birthing of our children.*

WATER DELIVERY AND BIRTH COMPLICATIONS

Water and Failure to Progress

As I noted in the previous chapter, "failure to progress" is often used as a reason for cesarean delivery. It is generally considered in obstetrical thinking that a woman should deliver within twenty-four hours. It is also considered a reason for intervention if a woman has "failed to progress" once she is in active labor—six centimeters or more—for two to four hours. First of all, laboring slowly is not abnormal. Many women have a latent labor pattern of three or four days. As long as the mother and baby are doing fine with strong vital signs, laboring over twenty-four hours or taking two to four hours to dilate a centimeter is not wrong. It is certainly no call for a cesarean section. Cohen and Estner state, "We know that failure to progress is seldom an issue at home births or at midwife-assisted births, and we contend that the mere idea of a time limit for delivery can be enough to cause labor dysfunction."[33]

If, during labor, dilation has slowed, many women find that getting in a warm bath or shower is just the helpful support they need to relax and allow themselves to go beyond the point where they want to stop. I feel that wanting labor to stop is an almost universal experience for women. It seems natural to me to have thoughts during labor like, "Okay, I've done this long enough. I think I'll stop now and go play tennis, do the laundry, and then I'll come back." Thoughts like these are an indication to me that the woman is expanding in her labor faster than her ego is willing to go along with at that time. *Often, "failure to progress" is simply the amount of time it takes to process through the thoughts and feelings of wanting to stop.*

Medical education does not prepare doctors to help a woman release psychological thoughts and feelings that may be preventing her from a continuous smooth flow in labor. If doctors, nurses, or midwives learn these abilities, it is usually not a result of their direct medical education but a development of their intuition through experience or accessing auxiliary educational programs in birth facilitation. This lack of awareness of a broad range of options in facilitating birth that I observed in the medical community caused me to want to develop educational programs that presented a wider range of options than were presented in standard obstetrical training. Many medical professionals are learning that having a good bedside manner can mean the difference between a labor progressing or failing to progress, between a patient moving forward in their healing or becoming more ill. Medical professionals are not just technicians but also can serve as a stimulus for people to awaken to their own healing abilities. My experience has shown me that the deeper I am willing to join with a laboring woman, the easier it is to facilitate a smooth, flowing birth. The ability to deeply connect with people requires as much development and learning as does learning the medical technology that is available to support birth.

If your labor is slowing down or "failing to progress" while laboring in warm water, you might try moving in a different way in the water, changing the temperature of the water, letting in some fresh air, getting out of the tub, taking a walk, or even going outside, if that is possible in your birthing environment. Often, a change in the external environment is a stimulus for a change in the internal environment. Water, being nonlinear, is a wonderful stimulus for helping a woman give up linear thinking about time and performance that often lies underneath "failure" to continue opening and dilating in birth.

Water, by its very nature, will not fail to progress. On the contrary, water will continue to progress and flow to the end of the boundaries of its container and then will overflow those boundaries when the source of the water is greater than the container. What an incredible metaphor for a birthing woman to connect with and to put her in a process that does continue to progress, one way or another, until the birth of the baby is complete. What solace there can be in our friend, the water, as you so willingly progress without failure!

Water and Cephalopelvic Disproportion

Cephalopelvic disproportion (CPD) is a term used to indicate that the baby's head or whole body (fetopelvic) is believed to be too large to fit through the mother's pelvis. Cohen and Estner report that CPD is given as the primary indication in one-third to one-half of all cesarean deliveries.[34] CPD is another catch-all reason given for cesarean sections when a doctor and birthing family do not trust that a woman's pelvis will soften, stretch, and open up to accommodate her baby's body, or that a baby's head will soften and mold itself to fit through the mother's pelvis. Cohen and Estner state, "The baby's size is only one of many factors that determine its ability to be born normally, and certainly not the most important factor. A determined mother and healthy pelvis can safely birth a healthy baby of almost any size." They go on to say, "Our success rates are much higher than in previous studies, with 85 to 90 percent of the women who have been sectioned for CPD going on to have VBACs (vaginal birth after cesarean), often with larger babies."[35]

If a laboring woman has warm water available to her and uses it at the first indication of someone being concerned about the size of her pelvis in relation to the size of her baby, she can often go deeply enough inside her own body and with her baby to allow themselves to stretch, open, and mold in just the right way for a perfect delivery. The same would also be true for a woman who had a previous cesarean based on CPD, like my friend Robbie Davis-Floyd, who, as described in the previous chapter, had a cesarean for failure to progress and CPD with a seven-pound baby, and later, a VBAC at home with a ten-pound baby. Laboring in warm water, as Robbie did on and off for three days, can put you in the perfect medium to help you melt away your anxiety and be in the moment in your process of labor and birth with your present baby.

Many women who might be diagnosed with CPD in a standard hospital setting never are because they choose birth settings— either home, birth center, or hospital—in which a wide range of support for a normal delivery is present. Settings that include not only the use of warm water but also little emphasis on time, performance, or having technology be dominant over the woman and her baby will also be settings in which CPD or failure to progress are not likely to occur.

The concern with CPD is "fit." Will the baby be too big for the mother's pelvis and the mother's pelvis too small? Certainly, the pelvic diameter can be widened by two-to-three centimeters if the mother gets on her hands and knees, in water or out. Yet underlying concern about fit is our underlying anxiety about nature. Can we trust that nature has given mothers and babies all the flexibility, stretchiness, and movement that they need to conform to one another's bodies in a perfect "passing through" motion? Or do we fear that somehow nature will go awry, and the baby will be stuck behind the mother's unopened doorway? Once again, water can be the perfect reminder to trust the flowing, harmonious fit of the container and the contained.

Water and Meconium

A baby's first poop is called meconium. It is "present in the intestine from about the sixteenth week of intra-uterine life. It is dark green/greenish-black in color, being composed of bile pigment, fatty acids, mucus and epithelial cells."[36] When it is thick, it looks much like tar. Ordinarily, a baby does not poop until sometime during its first twenty-four hours outside the womb. The presence of meconium staining in the amniotic fluids is usually considered as a sign of possible distress in the baby. Certainly, when coupled with raised, lowered, or erratic heart tones, it is seen as a sign of distress. Linda Church of the Family Birthing Center states, "When spontaneous rupture of membranes occurs while in the tub and meconium is present, the woman may be encouraged to get out of the tub so that the fetus may be further evaluated."[37] If there are no other signs of distress, the mother may safely return to the water for delivery.

Another concern when meconium is present is that the baby may inhale it during birth and contract meconium-induced pneumonia, which could be fatal. One midwife I interviewed attended a water delivery where the baby came out in amniotic fluid that had meconium. She felt it was beneficial that the baby came out underwater and was not stimulated to breathe in and possibly inhale meconium. Rather, the larger body of water diluted and washed away the meconium and the baby came up for air and breathed without any difficulty. I also attended a water delivery in which the bag of water ruptured at delivery with the presence of meconium; the baby did not inhale the meconium but came out of the water and began to breathe normally.

The mere presence of meconium is not an automatic indication not to have a water delivery, but it is an indication for further careful assessment physiologically and emotionally. If throughout labor and delivery, the birthing mother is encouraged to express her feelings through sound, movement, tears, talking, breathing, or any way she chooses to, she will be much less likely to have bottled-up stress, which contributes to the progress of the labor and to the baby's experience of stress in being born.

Pooping is the body's way to let go of substances that are not needed and, in fact, may be toxic. If a mother continually lets go of her feelings/thoughts that are not needed and may also be toxic if held onto, she will be providing a context for herself and her baby that release is natural, safe, and appropriate. In such a context, a baby could poop meconium or not without being in any undue stress.

Water and Elevated Blood Pressure

The midwifery textbook by Myles states that a woman in labor with a blood pressure of 130/80 should have the doctor notified "so that sedatives can be prescribed."[38] Linda Church reports on a study that found that women with high blood pressure were able to reduce their blood pressure by being immersed in warm water. About her own practice at the Family Birthing Center, Church adds, "We have noticed numerous times that an elevated blood pressure can be reduced dramatically within minutes of immersion in a heated pool of water."[39] Many women have told me that being in warm water helps take the pressure off, and this also seems to hold true with blood pressure. The calming and relaxing medium of water works to keep blood pressure in balance.

Water and Postpartum Hemorrhage

Postpartum hemorrhage (PPH) is severe bleeding within the first 24 hours after delivery of the placenta. The woman's blood flow is monitored after delivery of the placenta, and if she loses more than 500 ccs. (or two cups of blood) in five to thirty minutes, additional measures are called for. Average blood loss postpartum is less than two cups. Hemorrhaging can be caused by the retention of blood clots, pieces of placenta that are still adhered to the uterine wall, or a uterus that is slow to contract after birth. Myles comments on the most common cause of PPH; "If the woman is permitted to come into the third stage of labor with a full bladder, this inhibits proper placental separation, and as a result hemorrhage is liable to follow."[40] Measures to stop hemorrhaging range from manual stimulation of the uterus and the administration of Pitocin (a synthetic hormone used postpartum to cause the uterus to clamp down and stop bleeding) to manual removal of the blood clots and any remaining pieces of the placenta and blood transfusions. Most homebirth midwives, who are well trained to manage

PPH, carry Pitocin with them to stop it. But they may first try what homebirth midwife Janneli Miller calls "midwives' magical speech," in which the midwife places her hands on the mother's shoulders, looks her in the eyes, and firmly states, *"Stop bleeding now!"* Often, the mother's body responds to this command, and the bleeding stops. If that doesn't work, midwives may then administer the herb Shepherd's Purse and perform uterine massage and bimanual uterine compression, meaning that they push on the uterus from both sides with their hands. Like hospital practitioners, homebirth midwives are also trained in manual removal of the placenta – a last resort, as it is extremely painful for the mother. If blood transfusions are needed, the homebirth or birth center midwife will transport the mother to the hospital, often with an IV already in place to ready the mother for the transfusion.

About judging blood loss after a water delivery, midwife Beth Haber comments; "I've learned to judge the redness of the water, but I have not had to deal with a serious postpartum hemorrhage. I imagine if that happened, we would remove the mother from the tub for clear assessment."[41] Linda Church states, "In the absence of complications, the mother may remain in the water with her baby for a few minutes after birth to enhance bonding ... We believe that delivery of the placenta while the woman is seated on the edge of the tub minimizes the chances of intrauterine contamination with the bath water."[42]

It can safely take anywhere from a few minutes to thirty minutes for the placenta to deliver. In my three water births, I stayed immersed in the water, nursing my babies and bonding until I had more contractions and felt the placenta ready to deliver, which usually took fifteen to thirty minutes. When ready, I stood up and delivered the placenta into a bowl, and then sat down in the water again to continue bonding. If I had experienced excessive bleeding, I would have left the tub for further assessment of the situation. One midwife told me of a case where a woman was bleeding excessively, and the midwife felt that taking her from the warmth of the tub would have been too much of a shock at that time. She kept her warm in the tub, working with her uterus, which began to contract and stop the bleeding. Then, she moved the mother to a warm bed. Generally speaking, the first step would be to remove the woman from the tub for careful observation and support.

I have felt myself, and observed, that many times after a woman has birthed her baby and is in rapture with that new being, she can have a tendency to forget that the birth is not completely over. To have the baby on the outside seems enough. To have to think about birthing the placenta—also called the "afterbirth"—can feel like too much, especially if the woman experienced intense pain in labor and delivery. Mother Nature provides women with ten to thirty minutes prior to the birth of the placenta so the mom and baby can focus on bonding with each other. Frequently, just about the time nursing is well underway, contractions begin again, and the placenta is delivered.

Too often, doctors in busy hospitals have rushed the delivery of the placenta by pulling on the cord, which can break the cord and leave pieces of the placenta inside the uterus, and actually cause more hemorrhaging than if they had simply waited. This has especially afflicted our poverty populations of women on Medicaid, because hospitals generally only allow a certain amount of time in the delivery room for these patients.[43] The birth of the placenta is rushed, and many of these women hemorrhage. I have found that gently reminding the woman about the birth of the placenta and/or touching her uterus has usually been enough to stimulate its delivery.

Water Delivery and Infection

A concern in water delivery has been that the mother's uterus may become infected after delivery of the placenta. For this reason, Dr. Odent and Dr. Rosenthal both had the mother leave the pool just before expulsion of the placenta.[44] At the Family Birthing Center, Linda Church reported one minor infection in the 483 women who gave birth in the water between February 1985 and June 1, 1989,[45] and this is typical in other studies as well.[46] Dr. Odent had no cases of maternal infection in the several hundred water births at Pithiviers, France.

I have found the time after the delivery of the placenta to be a good one for the father/partner and baby to bond and play in the water while the mother is getting settled in a warm, cozy bed. I have gotten into a warm bath with my baby within the first three days after delivery and have had no infections. Those first few days after delivery continue to be a good time for the father and baby to have water play together until the mother feels that it is safe for her to return to the water as well. Thus far, there is no evidence that water delivery increases the risk of maternal infection when the mother leaves the tub with the expulsion of the placenta. Even when the mother returns to the tub after expelling the placenta, no greater increase of maternal infections has been reported. However, even though today, many thousands of women have labored and/or delivered in water, the number of water deliveries is small compared to land births, and more research needs to be done regarding staying in a tub of water after delivery of the placenta.

Most maternal infections occur because of the introduction of contaminated gloves and instruments into a woman's vagina and cervix during exams, especially after the amniotic sac has ruptured. It is strongly recommended that no unnecessary cervical exams be performed on birthing women, especially once their bag of water has broken. Not only does each exam increase the risk of infection, but also those exams are often painful and can easily disrupt the flow of the birth. Cervical exams during labor should only be performed when it is truly necessary to know the amount of dilation or at the mother's request, and, as I noted in Chapter 2, laboring in water can prevent or at least decrease the performance of unnecessary cervical exams. Again, there seems to be no greater risk of infection in a tub of warm water than in the air. Dr. Odent has told me that, occasionally, women at Pithiviers whose waters had ruptured in early labor would later enter the bath to labor or deliver their babies, and there was no incidence of infection.

I have found that the more hopeless, helpless, or disempowered I feel, the more vulnerable I am to infection and illness. The more I feel like a victim, the more likely I will be victimized. Physiologically, this is demonstrated by invading microorganisms that the body cannot fight off, increasing the danger of infection.

One advantage in home birth settings over hospital settings is that the woman and her baby are in their home environment of microorganisms with which they are compatible and less likely to be infected by. Hospitals are generally where sick people go, and thus are potential sites of contagion, especially so during the coronavirus pandemic. Since pregnancy is not an illness, many people argue that hospitals are not appropriate places for birth. There may be more risk of infection in a hospital setting than in the home or freestanding birth center.

It is my experience that the more a woman feels empowered in her pregnancy and birth, and the more she feels innocent and safe in being a sexual birthing woman, the less likely she will be to have any infection, illness, or other complication in pregnancy or delivery.

Water and Fetal Distress

Signs of fetal distress are determined by close monitoring of the heart rate of the baby in utero. The normal rate is between 120 and 160 beats per minute. An increase or decrease of twenty beats could be an early sign of distress.[47] The most common cause of fetal distress is hypoxia, or lack of oxygen. The most frequent sources of hypoxia in birth are the administration of drugs to the mother, which then pass through the placenta to the baby, decreasing the amount of oxygen flowing to the baby, and the lithotomy position, in which the mother is lying flat on her back, thereby depressing the large blood vessel carrying oxygenated blood to the baby.

In water deliveries, there is no administration of drugs. The warm water serves to give pain relief and in no way minimizes the amount of oxygen flowing to the baby. If the mother does wish for extra pain relief, she may be allowed to breathe in nitrous oxide, which is also a harmless method of pain relief that is entirely under the mother's control. Some hospitals have nitrous oxide available in labor rooms; it can also easily be installed next to the tub (see Figure 3.11). Also, in water-assisted deliveries, the mother is free to move in many positions and usually delivers the baby in an upright position that does not curtail the flow of oxygen to the baby.

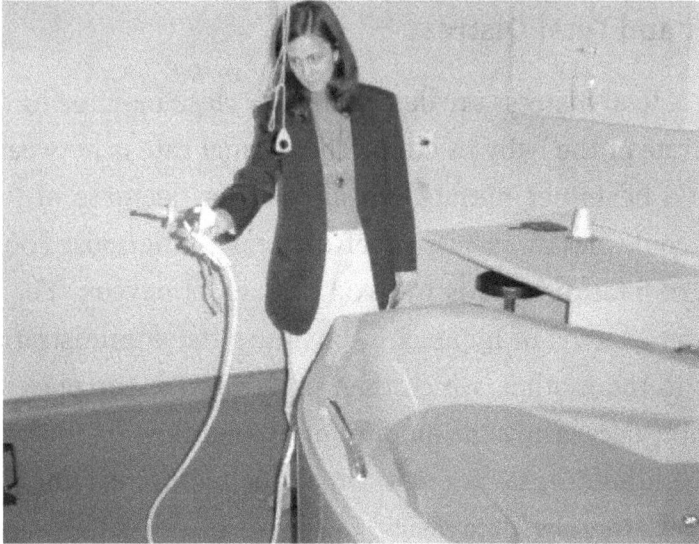

Figure 3.11. *A tub at St. Thomas Hospital, London, UK, with nitrous oxide installed and easily reachable. Photo by Robbie Davis-Floyd, used with permission.*

If there is cord compression at delivery, the baby's heart tones may drop momentarily. At such times, the birthing mother may be asked to breathe in pure oxygen until after the next contraction and release of the compression on the cord. Home, birth center, and hospital attendants have oxygen available in case it is needed. If there are signs of fetal distress in a water labor or delivery, the mother would most likely be asked to leave the tub for further assessment of her baby's condition. If all indications return to normal, she may again enter the tub for the delivery.

In pregnancies where the baby has been wanted by both parents, where there has been no demand that the baby be one sex over another, where the mother and baby have been strong and healthy during the pregnancy, and where the first stage of labor has flowed smoothly, there are rarely signs of fetal distress during delivery.

A birthing environment that is receptive and nurturing and a birth team that is connected with each other and the baby provide an environment that minimizes any stress to the baby. Delivery may be powerful work, intense and all-consuming, but not necessarily distressful or traumatic to the baby, who can experience her passage through the birth canal as a "gentle massage."[48]

Position of the Baby

I have only known of babies being delivered in the water in the regular, vertex/head-down position. I have heard of a doctor in Austria who has attended the deliveries of breech (bottom or feet first) and twins in water. I see no reason why breech, twins, or posterior (face up) presentations could not easily be delivered in water,[49] as long as there are no signs of distress in the mother or baby and the mother chooses to deliver in the water, and her birth attendant feels competent to assist such a delivery. Just as warm water can facilitate the more common presentation of a baby at delivery, it can also facilitate the less common presentations, which, in general, there is no need to classify as "high-risk."

Prematurity and Water Delivery

There have been no births of premature babies in water that I know of in the United States. Depending on the health of mother and baby and the degree of prematurity, there exists the possibility of delivering in warm water. Certainly, it would be easier on the premature newborn to enter the familiar element of water rather than dealing with direct gravity right away.

Igor Charkovsky and his wife had a premature daughter in the Soviet Union. The hospital doctors had given the baby up for dead. Charkovsky asked if he could take her home, and they said yes. He kept his daughter in a little pool of warm water, doing movement exercises with her for several months, and she both survived and thrived.[50]

It seems that such an idea holds possibility for premature babies. Some hospitals keep premature babies in the NICU on water beds and have reported excellent results. The use of water to assist premature infants both at delivery and postnatally is an area that needs further research. It makes sense that to continue their life in warm water, as they would have done in the womb, would support them to complete their growth and development.

Water and High-Risk Pregnancy

Women who have had diabetes or anemia during pregnancy, who have consistently smoked cigarettes or used drugs or alcohol, who have had inadequate or no prenatal care, who are anemic or have high blood pressure/pre-eclampsia, or who have had infections or other illnesses during pregnancy, are considered high risk. These women are the most likely to need the support of medical interventions and should consult their physicians and/or midwives regarding the appropriateness of using water in their labor or delivery.

The emotional-psychological conditions that give rise to these physical conditions must also be looked at as early as possible in the pregnancy. The number of children already in the family, the quality of the relationship between the mother and father/partner, the financial concerns of the family, if there have been previous miscarriages or abortions, or the recent death of a significant family member, the age of the mother and father, the mother's race, ethnicity, and socioeconomic status, religious beliefs about good and evil, beliefs about being a sexual woman and a mother – all of these can be extremely causal in setting up a foundation for a woman to be in a high-risk pregnancy situation.

Birth facilitators are trained to go deeply with a woman and her family into their own psyches to interweave their mental-emotional-spiritual selves with the real experience of physical pregnancy and birth. Symptoms that place women in the high risk category are messages connoting a cry for some kind of help. To fully support our birthing families, we need to supply them with this help and support them with good prenatal care.

It has often been noted that midwives, overall, spend more time with their patients than most obstetricians do. Midwives tend to be more intuitive and empathetic, and willing to address the emotional-psychological needs of their patients, as well as the physical. Doctors have told me that if they added emotional-psychological services to their prenatal care, the cost would be prohibitive. However, the amount of money that would not be spent on costly medical interventions would more than cover the cost of quality emotional-psychological services during pregnancy.

I feel it is time that we add trained birth facilitators—who are like doulas but have added skills, such as full-body massage and psychological therapeutic techniques—to our medical support teams for birthing families, and/or that nurses, midwives, and doctors become therapeutic facilitators as well as technical birth professionals.

I strongly recommend that women who are in any of the high-risk designations listed above seek help, not because they are wrong or bad, but because they are important human beings birthing other important human beings. There is rarely an obstacle so great that it cannot be resolved with a lot of willingness and loving support.

BENEFITS OF WATER BIRTH

◊ Water helps the mother merge the inner uterine environment with her outer environment.

◊ If a woman likes water, it is a pleasing environment for birth.

◊ Water is comfortable, offering ease of movement and flexibility of positions.

◊ Warm water helps the perineum to stretch without the need for warm oil or an episiotomy.

◊ Water provides relief from the pain of intense contractions.

◊ The warmth of water can be comforting to both the mother and baby.

◊ In water, the birthing woman feels weightless compared to gravity, so that the muscles do not have to work as hard to support the body.

◊ The energy saved in not being in a gravity environment can be used to go deeply within and connect with the baby.

◊ Water is a positive psychological cue for relaxation, and offers relaxation without drugs or medication.

◊ Water immersion decreases anxiety and increases natural oxytocin and endorphins, resulting in more rapid dilation.

◊ Being in water offers easy access to the baby's heart tones when the mother floats on her back, or wireless, waterproof telemetry can be used.

◊ The father/partner can be in the tub if desired and physically support the mother more easily than in gravity.

◊ Warm water is the familiar prenatal environment for infants and may help them transition more gently to extrauterine life.

- Any loud sounds are muffled, so the baby's hearing has a chance to adjust.

- Water birth is a way for women to symbolically and actually connect with Planet Earth, which is a predominantly water planet.

- Water birthing may be a way for birthing families to intuitively connect with cetaceans (whales and dolphins—the most intelligent species of our oceans) and may therefore help to bridge the gap between land and water, and the consciousness that each represents.

- Water facilitates the baby to release any stresses from the birth.

- Babies can easily learn to breathe while most of their body is submerged in the water so that breathing can be learned as a joyful experience rather than one of difficulty, hurry, or survival.

- Being born in water facilitates a baby to not inhale meconium, if present.

- Warm water reduces or balances elevated blood pressure.

RISKS OF WATER BIRTH

- Enforcing a water birth on a woman who does not choose it or who has a fear of water may produce negative results.

- Attempting a water birth without competent help or with no attendants present may not be wise.

- The baby could drown if not brought out of the water at the appropriate time.

- Water that is too hot may drain or tire the woman.

◊ If the woman's partner is not supportive of water delivery and the woman chooses to do it anyway, there would be a greater risk for complications.

◊ Possibility of infection, just as in dry or air/land birth.

◊ High-risk women may be at risk in water birth, just as they are in land birth, unless a competent birth attendant determines that there is a reason why water would support them more than a dry birth.

◊ Complications may develop from inexperienced birth attendants who thought they could support a water birth and discover in the process that they have fears or anxieties that then create a situation that frightens the mother and results in an unanticipated outcome.

◊ Just as in dry squatting deliveries, birth attendants do not have as easy access to controlling the delivery of the baby as they do when the woman is in the lithotomy position (on her back). Attendants must be more trustful of the mother and baby in their birthing process.

◊ If a woman is having twins, or the baby is in an unusual position—breech, posterior, or some variation—water delivery may not be recommended, since the mother may want her attendant to have easier access to assisting the delivery, and more intervention than usual may be necessary.

◊ If there are any indications of fetal distress, the birth attendant must evaluate whether water delivery is recommended.

PERSONAL STORIES ABOUT WATER AND BIRTH

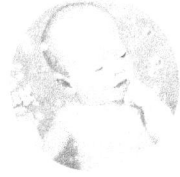

Mother's Account: Natalie's Birth
Portland, Oregon

by Irene Rae

I had my son Daniel, who's 11, by cesarean section and had a dreadful time. I wasn't planning on having a cesarean. My water broke in the middle of the night, and I went into the hospital and found out that he was breech. My doctor did not automatically plan for a cesarean but allowed me to go into labor to see what would happen. They prepped me and then wouldn't let me get out of bed. Essentially, I was left alone, waiting for my labor to start. My labor didn't start, so several hours later, they began to induce labor with Pitocin. Nothing happened for a long time. Finally, the Pitocin took effect, and when it did, it was a killer. I was in labor for thirteen hours. I was terrified. I had dilated only 3 centimeters. There was nobody there to talk to me. I didn't know what was going on. Finally, my doctor decided to do a cesarean. Now, I think being in the hospital, having residents coming in frequently to check my dilation, feeling alone, not getting to move around at all caused me to clamp down as tight as I could.

I was glad to be awake during the cesarean. When they took Daniel out, and I looked over at him in this little box next to me, I felt this enormous rush of emotion. I was thrilled. Tears were streaming down my face. But I didn't get to hold him and bond with him for a long time.

From the experience of Daniel's birth, I knew I wanted my next child's birth to be different. We happened to know a forward-thinking, holistic obstetrician in Portland. I knew he was the right person to talk to about being my doctor for this pregnancy because he acknowledged that how we birth our babies is important for the babies and the parents' psychological growth. Through this doctor and Dr. Michel Odent from France, we learned of birthing in water. I had been planning on a hospital birth. However, since no hospital in Portland would allow us to birth in water, we decided to have our baby at home. We felt that the element of water was important to have present in our birth.

The doctor introduced us to Phyllis Glickstein, a midwife who had done several water deliveries. I was worried she would not take me as a client, since having a previous cesarean delivery put me in a high-risk category. After interviewing us, she decided to work with us, and I am eternally grateful to her for midwifing us in our birth of Natalie.

The pregnancy went well. We were talking and bonding with the baby in the womb. We did rebirthing breathing sessions regularly. We even got our dream house on the Sandy River.

We were expecting her before Thanksgiving, so we had the tub prepared by the middle of October in case there was an early arrival. It's about three feet by seven feet. It's made of a wooden frame cut like a waterbed. It has a rim tacked around the top of it to sit on and two waterbed heaters and waterbed liners. We cleaned and rinsed it with chlorine and water. Then we filled it, let it warm up, and put salt in it. Since Natalie was born on November 26, we ended up draining and filling the tub a couple of times, just to have everything cleaned and prepared.

I had several false labors, and my midwife lovingly came out four times and went back home, no baby. Our doctor was in a car wreck shortly before the birth and had surgery. I said to him, "Nobody else knows how to deliver this baby. You've got to get well."

He made it to the birth, arm and leg in casts, and was a tremendous help. Having so many false alarms, I was beginning to worry; was I doing something wrong? Was the baby going to come out?

On a Monday morning, my husband Bill was going out the door on his way to go fishing. My water broke, and I said, "Wait, wait, come back. This is it! " We called Phyllis and the rest of our birth team. Phyllis came and walked with us up and down our beautiful driveway in the woods. It was wonderful. During the walk, I had dilated my first three centimeters. By the time we got in the house and into my bedroom, I had dilated up to five centimeters. When I heard that, I burst into tears and yelled, "I made it, I made it. I got past my three centimeters," which is where I had been stuck in Danny's birth. Feeling happy, I took a warm shower. When I got out, I felt like getting into our birth tub. Bill said when I sank down into the water, I just disappeared into a blissful Never Never Land.

As labor progressed, however, I went through a painful period when I began to have memories of being hit as a child. I was abused physically quite a bit, and those memories began flooding my mind as I progressed in labor. I had to breathe and yell and release a lot of anger that I felt. Shortly after this, I got out of the tub to have Phyllis check my dilation. I felt so uncomfortable out of the water that I couldn't wait to get back in. From that time on, I wouldn't get out again.

I felt like pushing and ended up pushing for two and one-half hours. Natalie was posterior—face up. A lip of my cervix was swollen. Bob reached inside me, arm in a cast, and held my cervix back so Natalie's head could get through. After that, she moved through quickly. My son Danny came in and sat right next to me, giving me the strength to push when I was afraid that she would never come out. Danny was right there with me, and we connected in a deep, beautiful way, beyond any words to describe.

I was in a squatting position most of the time when pushing. Then, I decided I wanted to be on my hands and knees. Bill was in front of me, and I had my arms around him, and Phyllis was behind me to catch the baby. I reached around when Natalie crowned, and I could feel her hair. At that point, the whole world changed. Suddenly, it was okay to be in pain; it was okay that everything was happening just the way it was. I knew I was alright, my baby was alright, and I could do whatever it took. There was a fusion that happened in me that allowed me to completely let go and relax.

I pushed her head out, face-up, and about three seconds later, her shoulders and then the rest of her body emerged. Bill said she just swam up to the top, arms and legs moving. I immediately flipped over, and she looked at me and Bill directly. We all smiled from the deepest part of our being. She was beautiful, and I assume we were beautiful to her. We brought her face up out of the water, she began to breathe, and I brought her to my breast for nursing. I was a little worried that she wasn't okay since her head was a little lumpy. Since Danny came out cesarean, he didn't look like that, and I had to be assured that she was fine. Her head had simply molded to fit through my pelvis and would shortly expand to its regular shape. When I felt some more contractions, I stood up and delivered the placenta in a bowl. Then Bill, Natalie, and I got in bed, and our friends came in and toasted us with champagne.

When our friends left the bedroom, we were alone for about an hour. I was lying with her. I looked at her, and she looked back at me, and it was like everything I had ever heard about this experience. Everything else in the universe disappeared except her eyes, and we connected for a long time.

For me, the important properties of the water were that it was warm, I could relax, and I could move. Being able to move was so fantastic. When I was five centimeters dilated until about nine centimeters, I actually almost swam back and forth in the pool. I was in constant motion during the contractions. I felt like I needed to be in those positions to let her wiggle around and get into the right position, and it lessened the pain when I was in the water. Since I was having a hard time relaxing my body, I could get on my knees in the water and reach around and feel if my perineum was relaxing. During each contraction, I'd put my hand on my thighs to help my mind and body merge into more relaxation. I couldn't have been in some of the positions I was in if I hadn't been in the water. The ability to move around in labor and pushing was the biggest support water provided for me.

After the birth and after emptying the tub, we kept it in our house for another three months until someone else needed it. It had a certain smell to it, possibly from the water liner. Every time I would go back into that room, I would smell that smell, and it just filled me with wonderful emotions and feelings. It was so positive to have a tub, to take responsibility for the preparation for it, and to be intimately familiar with it before I went into labor. After the birth, I *knew* that tub. It was my womb that helped me to do whatever I needed to do, to feel whatever I needed to feel to birth Natalie. I needed to release my feelings through sound and movement in Natalie's birth, and I don't think I would have been able to do that in a clinical setting.

I know the water was a good environment for Natalie too. She didn't cry. She came out relaxed and happy because she was born the way she wanted to be born. My water broke at noon, and I had her at 10:35 pm. She was nine pounds, and I didn't have any tears or stitches. None at all.

I also felt an extra measure of security in having both Phyllis and our doctor there. Phyllis has the ability to connect with birthing women that midwives do, and the doctor has the knowledge of allopathic medicine to use if needed. An ideal situation.

I think that because of the way we had Natalie, we're different parents than we would have been had we birthed in another way. It may be a chicken or egg kind of thing. Which comes first? Did we decide to have her that way because we decided we wanted to be a certain kind of parent, or are we now a certain kind of parent because we had her that way? Being as closely involved in the birth as we were, making sure everything was just so, there are now things in parenting Natalie that we make sure are just so. I don't know if we would have been so conscientious if we had done the birth another way. I had birthed Danny by cesarean in the hospital, bottle-fed him, and went back to work when he was two months old.

Now since I have had Natalie and learned how to bond, I have gone back with Danny, eleven years later, to recreate with him the same thing that happened with Natalie—holding him in my arms, long, relaxed eye to eye contact, and singing or making soothing sounds to him. Since he attended Natalie's birth and was a big help to me, he has greatly enjoyed getting to play baby again himself. He and I are now healing all of the incompletions and lack of bonding from that first birth experience.

There is no way I could parent Natalie the way I parented Danny at that time. I'm grateful Danny and I have bonded through Natalie's birth. Some children and parents, I know, will never experience that opportunity; they will have an unbonded birth experience, and that's the way it will stay. That's why it's so important to me to share my experience with other parents. It makes such a difference to have a gentle, loving, bonding birth experience right from the beginning. Certainly, we can re-bond and rebirth at any time, but why not let ourselves do it from the beginning? We need to take care of our moms. We need to take care of our dads. We need to take care of our babies. Doing so makes all the difference in the world – possibly the difference between peace and war, in ourselves, our communities, and our planet.

Father's Account: Natalie's Birth

by Bill Rea

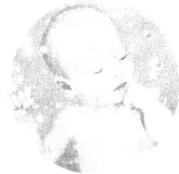

It made a big difference for me that we said that we wanted Natalie. This was our context before we even conceived Natalie. I knew I was responsible to this baby. We asked for her to come into our lives. I'd wake up and say to the baby in the womb and Irene, "Good morning, my miracles!" I felt connected.

Then, when I realized we were going to have her at home, I felt that I had to be even more responsible than I would if we were going to the hospital. I cared how the pregnancy was going, and every aspect of preparing for a birth at home became important to me. It was a thrill to be involved!

When Irene was in labor, I felt scared many times, worried that Irene would not be fine. There was pain to go through, and I stayed right with Irene and the baby through each contraction. I had fear, but I just kept putting out that everything would work out perfectly. I knew that in my own birth, my mother had managed to find a doctor who would allow her to birth without drugs. That was pretty innovative at the time. I now feel that my birth opened up possibilities for me to have Natalie without drugs, at home, in warm water. I am grateful to my mother for giving me that kind of drug-free birth.

It's clear to me the water was calming for Irene. The reports I had read that water can help the woman relax made sense to me. Whether someone wants to have their baby be born underwater or not, I'm sure that doing part of the labor in water is helpful to the mother. It takes away some of the aspects of weight and gravity, and lets the mother be in whatever position she wants. Water is therapeutic and helps the mother to relax, and that's important. There's nobody for whom I wouldn't recommend water labor.

In our case, it also worked well to have Natalie born in the water. I feel it helped her birth be gentler for her, and that's what we wanted for her. We didn't want our baby to have a lot of birth trauma that she would have to work through later on, that somehow might be a stop in her being as fulfilled a person as she could be. I know in our case, water helped us provide this for our child. There was something else about the birth—a quality that I can only call magical. When Natalie came out, she swam, or floated, up to the top, arms moving and eyes wide open, serene and peaceful. Such a miracle to behold!

An Imagined Baby's Account

by Rima Star

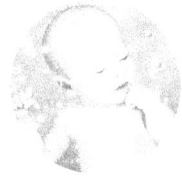

I felt like I had been in the womb a long time, and although I loved being inside my mother, I knew it was time to take my next step or swim, as was true in my case. Mother to me was warm and wet and wonderful. I had spent many hours swimming, rolling, and moving through her ocean, investigating every nook and cranny of her/me. I was especially happy when she would get into a large pool of water and swim or float and breathe for a long time. I loved the energy that flowed through my body when she did that. I could tell the difference when she was in the water. She would laugh and be more happy than usual and would always pay more attention to me, which I loved. I could even communicate to her, and most of the time, she knew what I was saying. It was at times like these that we were especially in tune with each other.

One day, I said to her, "Mom, when I come out of you, could I come out in the big water that you are in? I know I would like that!" She and my dad began to talk about this possibility and would swim and play in the water together and also do their breathing meditations in water. They began to envision just how it might feel to me to come out directly into warm water. They began to like the idea very much, and together, we created some beautiful visions for my water birth.

The more I grew, the more they grew emotionally and the more our mutual desire to birth in warm water at home grew. I felt excited, and I loved my parents for trusting me and my feelings about how I wanted to be born, even though they barely knew of anyone else who had birthed in this way. I felt so happy to know I would come out in warm water and be held by my mother that it gave me confidence and willingness to surrender to the birth process itself. When I felt that the time was near for me to swim out and be born, I was ready to go, excited and a little scared, but eager to begin my journey.

I felt warm rushes of energy begin to move through my mother and me, like big waves that would press against me and then release. My head moved down into my mother's pelvis, and I could feel the opening of her cervix become more and more mushy and soft each time a wave would come and push me against it. I became afraid as waves seemed to come faster and faster, and then I felt my mother put her hands over me and tell me I was doing perfectly, and I was safe. She told me that, together, she would open her body and I would move through her, and soon I would be in her arms and seeing her face to face. That was just the reminder I needed to relax and go with the flow. I also seem to recall that about the same time, I heard my dad tell my mother much the same thing that she had told me. It felt good to know that we were both so supported in our birthing journey. I felt my confidence in myself and my mother renewed.

There was a time when I felt my mother step into a tub of warm water. I could tell because sounds became more muffled, and she began to move around in ways she had not done before. She could kick her legs, roll over, and stretch. This felt good to me too, because I could stretch a little more when she did. I could also feel some new kinds of energy rushing through us that seemed to cause my thoughts to disappear, and I surrendered to a rhythmical dance of energy and emotions moving me, pressing and releasing over and over – a harmonious flow of pleasure. I could feel my mother's cervix not only soften but expand, and I could sense that soon my whole head would move through and into the birth canal.

My mother began to make low and long sounds that added vibrations to our birth dance. The sounds helped her and me to focus more intently on moving me through the birth canal. I could sense the tunnel passageway I was moving through and the open water beyond. What excitement! I knew there was no turning back now.

Suddenly, the soft bag of waters that had been cradling my head burst, and I felt my head slide into direct contact with my mother's skin in the tunnel and the warm water of the tub. What a rush of energy! I knew it wouldn't be long now.

My mother then began to push with the energy rushes and with me. She moved into some different positions, and I learned later that when I came out, she was on her hands and knees with my father behind her. One time she reached down and touched the top of my head as I began to peek through her opening. I felt so ecstatic when she touched me that I laughed and cried at the same time. I think she did too. The next thing I knew, my head was completely out, and my mother was stroking my face. I turned to one side, and the rest of me came out too. There was so much space, but my mother and our midwife were there to hold me, and I could float too. I just relaxed and felt that I had just come into a gigantic ocean of my mother's love. My mother must be big to have oceans inside of her and outside of her too. My mother's love was everywhere, outside as well as inside. Thank you, Mom, for birthing me into more of you. What an ecstatic surprise!

Next, I opened my eyes and saw my mother and father looking directly into me and felt another rush of laughing/crying joy. They were so beautiful. I knew I wanted to be closer, right next to my mother's heart. She knew this too and gently lifted my head out of the liquid ocean love, reminding me that the air was there to nurture me as the water had done. She held me close to her, and I could hear the familiar beating of her heart and feel the silken skin of her breast with my fingers – such exquisite sensations.

I began to experiment with breathing air in and out through my nose. It felt kind of tickly and fun. Then, I felt my lungs expand, and I opened my mouth and took a big, full breath. My body felt electric with energy and warmth and vibration. I was amazed I could do such a thing on my own, with my very own breath. I felt powerful and full of life. I settled into a rhythm of breathing and feeling warm, snuggled in my mother's arms with the warm water of the tub lapping around my body.

I became aware of the wetness of my mother's breast and a desire to taste her. I turned my head and, with my mouth, found her nipple and began to suckle. It was a surprise to discover that I could suckle and breathe at the same time. Soon, warm nectar came out of my mother's breast that tasted like the sweetness of Heaven. It flowed down into my stomach, and I entered into deep relaxation. I fell asleep, my father singing lullabies to me and my mother rocking me securely against her breast.

Birth Attendant's Account:
Alexander's Birth, September 12, 1988
(Moscow, Soviet Union)

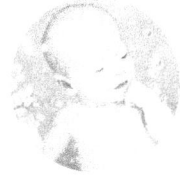

by Rima Star

I did not realize in 1979 when I saw the water babies of Igor Charkovsky swimming across my TV screen that I would one day find myself in the Soviet Union attending a birth with this unusual man. I also did not know, when I saw those babies scooting by, smiling underwater, that I would find myself pregnant in the next year with my first baby since the accidental drowning of my 4-year-old son in 1972.

The impression those joyous water babies made on me in those brief moments on television was deep and profound. It began to awaken in me a memory that there was indeed a way for both mothers and babies to be playful and have joy in this most significant life transition of birth and parenting.

After the devastating loss of my son to water in 1972, it was indeed a miracle that I was able to even see the possibility of water as a place of pleasure, safety, and bonding for mothers and babies. Nevertheless, my husband and I, with the assistance of midwives and friends, birthed our daughter Mela Noel on November 5, 1980, into a tub of warm water. It was a beautiful birth. Although we had only known one other couple who had birthed their baby in water, we felt confirmation in the fulfillment we had in our experience that our choice had been correct for us and for Mela.

After eight years and two more water births, I found myself on a plane for the Soviet Union. Orien Margaret Star was born on August 1, 1984, and Hank Lee Star was born on May 6,

1987. Both were amazingly ecstatic births, each with a deeper appreciation of the superfluid motion and warmth of water. I experienced being in water as being immersed in liquid love.

I had also attended sixty other births, lectured across the United States, and written a book, *The Healing Power of Birth* (1986), to share the incredible transformations I had experienced through birth.

When my friend and Mela's godmother, Sondra Ray (author of *Ideal Birth*), called and said she was arranging a trip to the Soviet Union to meet Igor Charkovsky and Soviet midwives, I did not even hesitate to say, "Yes, I will go." It seemed that the time was right for me to go and express my gratitude to Charkovsky, Soviet midwives, parents, and babies for opening up new possibilities in birth.

I had managed to see several film clips, read occasional articles on Soviet water babies, and read the book *Water Babies* by Swedish author Erik Sidenbladh on Igor's life and work. I knew that people from around the world had been drawn to go to the Soviet Union to meet the man himself (now deceased) and learn firsthand what he was doing and why.

I felt the same way as I reflected on what I knew about his work. I knew he had saved his own premature daughter's life in the early 1960s, when the doctors and hospitals had given her up to die, by keeping her in water and doing movement exercises with her. She is now a healthy adult. After his success with his own daughter, doctors and parents would bring him other premature or traumatized infants to see if his magic would work with them. It did, and his reputation began to grow. He began working with healthy children in water, as well as experimenting with the possibility of birthing in water by training cats and other animals to swim and birth in water. He reasoned that since babies grow and develop in water for nine months, being born in water would be a familiar and gentle introduction into a new and stimulating environment. He also felt the weightlessness of water would support the infants' brains in a way that would allow for optimal brain development in the critical first moments after birth.

I knew that this man was deeply committed to enabling our children to realize their fullest potential, and I was excited to be meeting him myself. Just knowing what he was doing in the Soviet Union helped give me confidence in pursuing my work with pregnant women and birth in the United States.

We flew into Helsinki, Finland, and took an overnight train to Moscow. Crossing the barbed wire borders with their armed guards brought up countless images from the 1950s elementary school scares of the Soviet monolith. However, when I looked into the faces of the young soldiers who examined our passports, all I could see was the fresh innocence of hearts, desiring, just as I was, to correct the images of "enemy" that each of our countries had painted for us.

Our group of eighteen travelers arrived at our Moscow hotel in time to hear that we were invited to come immediately to an apartment complex where Soviet TV was filming Igor and his water babies. We arrived and were greeted by a large group of excited Soviet parents, midwives, children, and Igor himself. He immediately walked up to my friends Karen and Charles Glueck and their two children, David, age 2, and Christopher, age 2 months. He wanted to know, "Are these American water babies?" Upon hearing "Yes," he asked if he could swim Christopher with the Soviet water babies who were swimming in the Plexiglas tank beside where we were standing. Igor undressed Christopher, connecting with him, while Karen asked her son if he wanted to swim. His smile and curiosity told us yes. Igor then put Christopher's feet in the palm of one hand and, holding Christopher's hand in the other, lifted him up in the air. Then, he lowered Christopher into the water, dipping him under and up with the other little baby in the tank while Soviet camera crews filmed.

Also in attendance that day was John Lilly, the well-known dolphin researcher from America. He was obviously delighted to see these American and Soviet water babies swimming as happily in their water environment as dolphins do in theirs. He said, "If babies can be born into the world playing the way dolphins do, humanity stands a chance of making it."

Having completed his swim, Christopher was bundled up in his mother's arms, happily falling asleep. The Soviet camera crews were putting up their equipment while radiant Soviets and Americans began to hug and talk earnestly about their mutual desire for happy, healthy babies that cared to create peace in the world and not war. In this atmosphere of enthusiasm, Igor received a phone call and excitedly came back to ask if Sondra, myself, Kate (a midwife from Atlanta), and Diane (a midwife from Australia), would like to attend a water birth that was about to happen. We, of course, were thrilled! For Sondra, Kate, and Diane, it was the first water birth they had attended. For me, it was a dream come true to connect with a real Soviet family who was birthing their child in water as I had done.

Igor, his midwifery partner, Alya, myself, and Sondra rode in a cab for almost an hour to arrive in the early evening at a flat in a large apartment complex in Moscow. We entered the flat with our hearts opening to the wonder and mystery of the birth we were about to experience. The two-bedroom flat was rich with excitement and love. An elated and expectant father met us at the door, his two sons beaming on either side of him. They knew their newest brother or sister was about to be born. A friend was in the dining room, playing the piano and singing. Her melodious tones floated into the bathroom, where a radiant birthing mother was squatting in the bathtub being attended by two midwives as she moaned and breathed past her last thoughts of impossibility.

Her face lit up when she saw Igor and Alya, and she smiled a greeting to each of the four of us as we connected with her at the doorway of the bathroom. Her energy shifted as Igor and Alya began to work with her and the baby, moving their hands in circular motions about eight inches above her belly. They were working with the etheric body just as one might massage the physical body. In fact, working with the etheric body seems to facilitate the physical body to open up. I call this "smoothing the aura or energy field of the mother and baby." They were creating a matrix of safety for the mother to feel supported in letting go and delivering her baby into the world outside her womb.

There was much excitement as the woman gave a push, and out into the water came a black-haired, large, and beautiful boy. He remained underwater for a few seconds as Igor slipped the cord from around his shoulder. Then the baby was lifted out of the water into his mother's arms. The dad and brothers were kneeling by the tub in awe and gratitude towards the mother and thrilled with the newest member of their family.

Then Igor did something that surprised both Sondra and me but did not seem to surprise the mother or baby. He took a pan of cold water and poured it over both of them; neither one seemed to mind. I thought, perhaps, he did it because the baby was a little blue or to prevent the mother from going into shock. I later learned that the use of cold water at birth was common in

Russia. It is believed a dip in icy water sets a strong constitution and immune system. We learned from Alya that members of her Family Health Clubs cut holes in ice in winter and dip babies, children, and adults for their good health.

After this cold-water splash, Igor held the baby and dipped him up and under the warm water. The placenta was still inside the mother, and the cord was attached to the baby. The mother then held the baby to her breast as he looked around, connecting and bonding to his new environment. Since the birth of the placenta did not seem imminent, we helped the mother and baby into the bedroom, where they could snuggle and we could help her to birth the placenta.

The mother was excited with her new baby and with our presence at her birthing. She wanted Sondra and me to know that she had read our books, which had been translated and written by hand in Russian, and which Igor and the midwives gave to each pregnant couple to read prior to their birthing. We had no idea this had been happening and felt honored to be supporting Russian birthing in this way. One of the things that amazed me was that at this time, Russians had no access to copy machines, so translated copies of American books were precious to them.

I was happy to connect with the mother, and felt that she had temporarily forgotten to birth the placenta in her enthusiasm to communicate with us. I walked out of the bedroom and into the kitchen to bring her something to drink. One of the Soviet midwives quietly came up to me and asked, "What do you do in America for retained placenta?" I began telling her some of the things we do, from nipple stimulation to herbs, to channeling energy through the hands, to manual removal of the placenta, which of course, we try to avoid because it is so painful for the mother.

I learned that abortion was one of the most common forms of birth control in the Soviet Union and women had, on average, seven or eight abortions during their childbearing years. Frequent abortions may leave scar tissue in the uterus, which could account for difficulties in releasing the placenta.

We returned to the bedroom to find the mother and baby happily nursing. The father, who had been preparing caviar, and the two sons, who had been laughing and playing with the guests, returned also. The rest of us left the room so the new family would have privacy to bond. She was having no further contractions.

In the living room, we began discussing our experiences with birth and the status of midwifery in both countries. Yet, we all felt an underlying concern about the birthing of the placenta, and soon, we returned to the bedroom to see how things were progressing. The woman still was not having contractions. The father and sons left the room, and we encircled the mother and baby to focus on the placenta coming out. I asked her if I could lay my hands on her uterus, and while I did, the Soviet midwives began to give her visualizations of having contractions and birthing the placenta. Our circle of women generated a warm glow of love as Russian and English words were quietly exchanged back and forth. There was a hum to the silence as midwives from two sides of the globe united in a mutual effort of support. Soon, the mother began to have contractions. Suddenly, Igor walked into the room at about the same time and asked the mother to return to the bathtub. While Dad held the baby, Mom squatted in the tub. Igor poured a bucket of cold water over her, and moments later, the placenta was birthed. There was much jubilation as we helped the mother dry off and return to the bedroom.

Shortly afterward, as I was talking with friends in the living room, one of the Soviet midwives came up to me again. This time, she was carrying some rather thick suturing material and a needle. She asked, "Would you sew up the woman? She has a tear, and it is illegal for us to do it." I replied that I had not done suturing, but a midwife with our group had. I found Kate, and together, we went to see what we could do. The mother was excited about having the tear repaired, for she knew if we did not do it, she would have to heal without the benefit of suturing. I held a flashlight as we examined the mother to determine how many and where she needed stitches. Kate prepared a sterile field; two Soviet midwives sat on either side of the mother holding her hands and translating what Kate was telling her about the procedure she would be doing. We also held acupressure points to numb the sensation in that area. Six stitches were finally completed after stopping and starting many times. The mother breathed through the pain and said that it was not too bad at all. I was thankful that the natural endorphins in her body from the birth were still present to lessen the sensation of pain.

Everyone breathed a sign of gratitude as we basked in the glow of our mutual love and support. Something truly momentous had happened. Not only did we merge people from enemy countries in support of this new life, but we also merged what could be thought of as "enemy" technologies of home birth and medicine. Old categories of belief slipped away as we stepped out into the uncharted territory of the heart.

With the birth complete, everyone joined together as the proud papa brought out caviar and opened bottles of champagne to celebrate. There was profuse toasting for the new baby, the mother, the Americans, the Soviets, and for peaceful births throughout the world. Songs were sung in Russian and English.

Suddenly, I noticed we were no longer translating back and forth but communicating directly in animated voices, our respective languages no longer seeming to be a barrier to us.

The father and the sons began to take beautiful blue and white pottery from their shelves to give to us as gifts, as we were giving gifts of postcards and cassette tapes to the boys and other gifts to the baby and mom. One of the most important exchanges came when Kate gave her fetoscope to Alya, Igor's midwifery partner and founder of the Family Health Clubs in Moscow. None of the Soviet midwives had fetoscopes, and it was a thrill to see Alya joyfully receive this gift. They all expressed desires to receive equipment and to be trained to use it in support of their home births in Moscow.

During the remainder of the toasting, Alya sat at the dining room table, quietly writing. Then she announced she had one final toast to make, in the form of her "Declaration on the Human Right to Freedom of Birth." Here, I offer this declaration to you and invite your alignment with the goal that all parents and children of Earth have the freedom to choose the birth atmosphere and support they most desire.

DECLARATION ON THE HUMAN RIGHT TO FREEDOM OF BIRTH

We, the undersigned alternative midwives of the Soviet Union, USA, United Kingdom, and Australia, having jointly assisted in the water birth of a new human being, baby Alexander, who has emerged in the Russian family of Klimous in the presence of his father and his brothers, appeal to the governments of all countries of the world, to all the doctors, healers, and midwives of any kind, to all circles of world society, to every woman and every man on our planet.

We claim the right of a human being to choose freely a time, a place, surroundings, and a way of his/her own birth, which is defined by the free will, preferences, and responsibility of his/her parents.

Thus, we claim the mother's and father's right to create the environment and to choose the way of their baby's birth.

We are convinced that a free, non-violent, natural, and soft birth delivery is the way to the creation of human beings marked with love, dignity, and health and open to their limitless spiritual power.

In free birth, full of love, openness, and high consciousness, we see the hope of a new world rising, a world free of violence, wars, aggression, hate.

In free birth, we see the way towards the birth of a new ecological consciousness, the expanding of human spiritual potential, and the rebirth of the human species.

Having taken part in the wonderful mystery and the joyful family celebration that united people from opposite continents, we appeal to the people of the whole world to create the human right of free birth on our planet. We want to have the opportunity, confirm the right, and call all midwives of the world to deliver together newborns of different countries in the presence of relatives and friends, to prepare fathers and mothers for the free and conscious birth of their own children, and to use freely, exchange, and multiply their unique experience of non-violent birth.

In the basic human right of free birth, we see the hope of survival for humanity, the hope of saving the life of our planet.

Endnotes

1   Jackson et al, "Incorporating Water Birth into Nurse-Midwifery Practice," *Journal of Nurse-Midwifery*, Vol. 34, No. 4, July/August, 1989, pp. 196-197.

2   Church, Linda K., "Water Birth: One Birthing Center's Observations," *Journal of Nurse-Midwifery*, Vol. 34, No. 4, July/August, 1989, pp. 165-166.

3   Meenan AL, IM Gaskin, P Hunt, et al. 1991. "A New (Old) Maneuver for the Management of Shoulder Dystocia." *Journal of Family Practice* 32(6):625-629.

4   Personal interview with Dr. Bastyr, Seattle, 1985.

5   Ozhiganova, Anna, "The Birth of a New Human Being: The Utopian Project of the Late Soviet Water Birth Movement and Its Inheritors." In *Birthing Techno-Sapiens: Human-Technology Co-Evolution and the Future of Reproduction*, edited by Robbie Davis-Floyd. London: Routledge, 2021, pp.

6   See: Cheyney, Melissa, Marit Bovbjerg, Courtney Everson, *et al.* 2014. "Outcomes of Care for 16,924 Planned Home Births in the United States: The Midwives Alliance of North America Statistics Project, 2004 to 2009." *Journal of Midwifery & Women's Health* 59 (1): 17-27; de Jonge, A. et al. 2009. "Perinatal Mortality and Morbidity in a Nationwide Cohort of 529,688 Low-Risk Planned Home and Hospital Births. *BJOG: An International Journal of Obstetrics and Gynecology* 116 (9):1177-1184. DOI: 10.1111/j,1471-0528.2009.02175.x/full; de Jonge, A. et al. 2015. "Perinatal Mortality and Morbidity up to 28 days after birth among 743,070 Low-Risk Planned Home and Hospital Births: A Cohort Study Based on Three Merged National Perinatal Databases. *BJOG: An International Journal of Obstetrics and Gynecology* 122(5):720-728;

Stapleton, Susan Rutledge, Cara Osborne, and Jessica Illuzzi. 2013. "Outcomes of Care in Birth Centers: Demonstration of a Durable Model." *Journal of Midwifery & Women's Health* 58 (1): 3-14.

7   Dekker, Rebecca. "The Evidence on Water Birth." 2018. Found at: Evidence on Waterbirth (evidencebasedbirth.com)

8   Jackson et al., pp. 195-196.

9   Jackson et al., p. 193.

10 Odent, Michel, *Primal Health*, London: Century Hutchinson, Ltd. , 1986, p. 12.

11 Jackson et al., p. 195

12 Jackson, et. Al., p. 196

13 Myles, op. cit., pp. 320-321.

14 Jackson et al., p. 194.

15 Church, op. cit., p. 169.

16 Jackson, et. al., p.195.

17 Jackson, et. al., p. 194.

18 Cheyney M, M Bovbjerg, C Everson, W Gordon, D Hannibal, S Vedam. 2014. "Outcomes of Care for 16,924 Planned Homebirths in the United States: The Midwives Alliance of North America Statistics Project, 2004 to 2009." *Journal of Midwifery & Women's Health* 59(1):17-27.

19 Gregory Elizabeth C.W., Patrick Drake, and Joyce A. Martin. 2018. "Lack of Change in Perinatal Mortality in the United States, 2014–2016." NCHS Data Brief No. 316. https://www.cdc.gov/nchs/data/databriefs/db316.pdf; Davis DA. 2019a. "Obstetric Racism: The Racial Politics of Pregnancy, Labor, and Birthing." *Medical Anthropology* 38(7):560-573. doi.org/10.1080/01459740.2018.1549389. Davis DA. 2019b. *Reproductive Injustice: Racism, Pregnancy, and Premature Birth*. New York: New York University Press.

20 Cohen, Nancy Wainer, and Lois Estner. 1983. *Silent Knife: Cesarean Prevention and Vaginal Birth after Cesarean*. South Hadley, Mass: Bergin and Garvey Publishers, Inc., p. 18. Cohen and Estner 1983, p. 19.

21 Davis-Floyd, Robbie. *Birth as an American Rite of Passage*, 3rd edition, Abingdon, Oxon: Routledge, 2022.

22 Cohen and Estner, p. 8

23 Davis-Floyd, Robbie. *Birth as an American Rite of Passage*, 3rd edition, 2022.

24 Cohen and Estner, p. 9

25 Odent, Michel, *Birth Reborn*. New York: Random House, 1984, p. 16, and also in the

BBC Documentary film, *Birth Reborn*.

26 Davis-Floyd, Robbie, "The Technological Model of Birth," *Journal of American Folklore* 100 (398):491-492, 1987.

27 Davis-Floyd, Robbie, in Star, Rima, *The Healing Power of Birth*, Austin, Texas: Star Publishing, see "Oppositional Paradigms," p. 120.

28 Davis-Floyd, Robbie. 1994. "The Technocratic Body: American Childbirth as Cultural Expression," *Social Science and Medicine* 38(8):1125-1140.

29 Davis-Floyd, Robbie, in Star, Rima, *The Healing Power of Birth*, pp. 129-130.

30 Davis-Floyd, Robbie, in Star, Rima, *The Healing Power of Birth*, pp. 129-130.

31 Odent, Michel, *Birth Reborn*, p. 46

32 Odent, Michel, *Birth Reborn*, p. 46

33 Cohen and Estner, p. 191

34 Cohen and Estner, p. 17

35 Cohen and Estner, p. 98

36 Myles, Margaret F., *Textbook for Midwives*, London: Churchill/Livingston, 1981, p. 483.

37 Church, Linda K., p. 167.

38 Myles, p. 276

39 Church, p. 176

40 Myles, p. 423

41 Jackson et al, p. 197

42 Church, p. 168

43 For a description of the mistreatment of women on Medicaid and members of marginalized groups, see Davis-Floyd, Robbie, *Birth as an American Rite of Passage*, 3rd edition. Abingdon, Oxon: Routledge, 2022.

44 Odent, Michel, *The Lancet*, December, 1983, p. 1476 and Rosenthal in Church, p. 168

45 Church, p.165

46 See "Water Birth: Benefits, Risks, Costs, What to Expect, and More" (healthline.com)

47 Myles, p. 301

48 Sheila Kitzinger, 1983. Keynote presentation at the first-ever conference of the Pre- and Perinatal Psychology Association of North America (PPPANA)—now known as APPPAH—the Association of Pre- and Perinatal Psychology and Health.

49 See Kamayani DC. 1989. "Water Birth: A European Perspective" *Journal of Midwifery and Women's Health* 34(4):190-192. https://doi.org/10.1016/0091-2182(89)90080-3

50 Sidenbladh, Erik, *Water Babies*, New York: St. Martin's Press, 1982, p. 56.

Chapter 4

WATER AND BONDING

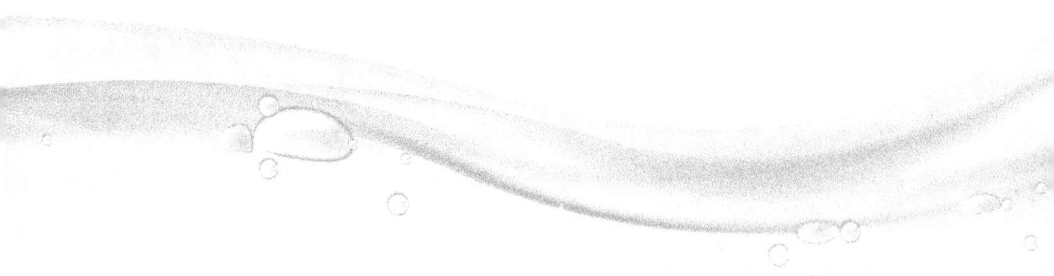

WHAT IS BONDING?

Webster's Dictionary defines the verb "to bond" as: *"To cause to adhere firmly; to embed in a matrix; to hold together or solidify; cohere."* Bonding is defined as, *"The formation of a close personal relationship (as between a mother and child) especially through frequent or close association."*[1]

Klaus and Kennell further define bonding:

> By general consensus, the term 'bond' refers to a tie from parent to infant, whereas the word "attachment" refers to the tie in the opposite direction from infant to parent...a bond can be defined as a unique relationship between two people that is specific and endures through time...we have taken as indicators of this attachment the attachment behaviors of fondling, kissing, cuddling, and prolonged gazing—behaviors that serve both to maintain contact and to exhibit affection toward a particular individual...Strong attachments can persist during long separations of time

and distance, even though often there may be no visible signs of their existence. Nonetheless, a call for help even after 40 years will bring a mother to her child and evoke attachment behaviors equal in strength to those in the first year of life.[2]

Klaus and Kennell, in asking the question when a parent's love of their baby begins in relation to the sensitive period after birth, report on a study that asked, "When did you first feel love for your baby?" The results: "During pregnancy, 41%; at birth, 24%; first week, 27%; and after the first week, 8%." They further state, "The onset of this maternal affection after childbirth was more likely to be delayed if the membranes were ruptured artificially, if the labor was painful, or they had been given a generous dose of meperidine (Demerol)."[3]

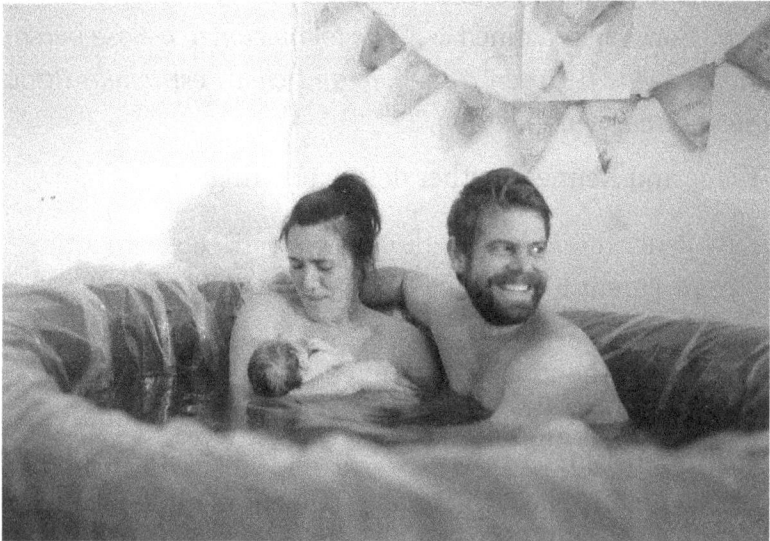

Figure 4.1. *My daughter Orien bonds in water with her first baby Josie, while her husband Andy gives a celebratory smile to the midwife. Photograph by Monet Nicole, used with permission.*

One of the primary reasons researchers became interested in this sensitive period after birth was when hospital staff observed that premature babies who had been sent home thriving "would sometimes return to the emergency rooms abused by their parents or failing to thrive without organic disease." However, when these infants were returned to the hospital, they would once again thrive. This information tells us that these infants felt bonded and secure in the hospital with hospital staff and not in their homes with their parents.[4]

Separation and other maladies that occur after birth can result in dysfunctional parenting. These dysfunctions can range from the extreme of the battered child to parenting from duty or obligation with no feeling of attachment or love. That is why it behooves you as a parent to examine your background in regard to bonding and infancy with your parents, as well as with other caregivers. If you can come to resolution and peace with these experiences, you will begin your parenting of your infant from a strong foundation of functionality and wholeness, and if you continue to examine your relationship to your parents, as you observe your response to parenting your infant, you will embark upon a rich, rewarding, and joyful parenting experience. Most people feel so abandoned and unbonded themselves that it is difficult to give to their child what they themselves do not feel they have. This is one reason myself and others offer "preparation for parenting" workshops to heal the unbonded infant and child within, so that we as adults can give our children the best we have to offer.

Regarding an interesting study by Poindron and Le Neindre on bonding behavior with sheep, Klaus and Kennell report, "If separation begins at birth and lasts for four hours, 50% of the ewes are still willing to accept lambs. However, when a separation beginning at birth lasts for 12 to 24 hours, the percentage of ewes willing to accept lambs drops to 25%. In contrast, if a 24-hour separation does not begin until 2 to 4 days after birth, all ewes will accept their lambs."[5] Another related study showed that blood plasma taken from a new mother rat within twenty-four hours after birth and injected into a non-mother rat induced maternal behaviors. However, blood taken just prior to the twenty-four-hour period and just after the twenty-four-hour period did not.[6] These studies point to the crucial importance of the bonding process in the first twenty-four hours after birth.

Klaus and Kennell report, "... in most [traditional] societies, the mother and baby are placed together with support, protection, and isolation for at least seven days after birth. The provision of food, wood, and water and a private time for the mother and infant to get to know each other are common in most cultures."[7] Such a practice seems so simple and yet so foreign to the experience of most babies in Western culture. When we consider the potential damage we do to our children and parents with standard procedures of separation after birth—which today are rarer in the U. S., where "rooming-in" is now more common, yet are still prevalent in many other countries—it is no wonder that some parents take whatever measures they need to be sure they will not be stopped or interrupted in their process of bonding with their newborn. This is one of the main reasons many parents choose home birth. The fact that you are reading this book already indicates to me that you have a high commitment to bonding with your newborn. However, it is important for you to be aware of the standard procedures in your hospital regarding mother-baby togetherness or separation after birth. If that hospital is behind the times and still separates mothers and babies for a period of time after birth, you may want to look for a different hospital that offers 24/7 rooming-in. It is good to be aware of the overall condition of birth and bonding in our culture and to take action when and where we can to support all parents to bond with their newborns and children.

The ability to be close and to attach immediately after birth and continuing in infancy—called the "external gestation" period—sets a foundation for all further relationships in life. The mother-baby bond is the formative relationship from which the baby imprints what to expect in further relationships in childhood, adolescence, and adulthood. The quality and character of this first relationship with, primarily, the mother but also the father/partner and siblings, sets the stage for the quality and character of this person's future relationships. This is a time in which the infant needs to learn healthy dependency. It is important for babies to learn that they can, indeed, depend on their primary physical universe (the mother) to respond appropriately to her communications, and for the mother to learn the same about her infant. Not only does each respond appropriately to the other, but both do so with the feeling of love. Some of the most beautiful sculptures and paintings in the world are of the blissful beauty of the glowing relationship between the mother and the infant.

Some researchers call these first few hours after birth a "critical period," defined as a relatively brief time in which major changes in brain organization occur, and following which further change is difficult.[8] This definition has been used mainly to apply to physiological processes. However, it is not farfetched to apply it to the physical and emotional process of bonding in the first hours after birth. In my work with adults who have recalled major traumas in their lives as avenues for opening up their ability to love as adults, the trauma of separation from the mother immediately after birth is one of the most frequently recalled events. The statements people make when they are recalling one of these events have a finality about them: "I feel like I have lost the chance to connect with people. Where is my mother? Where is someone who can recognize, see, and hear me? What have I done wrong to be taken from my mother? I must need to be separate from my mother to survive. I am sad that I have to be separated rather than connected to survive in this place. I wish I were back in the womb and close to my mother."

Even when these babies–most of us of the Baby Boom (1946-1964) and Gen-X (1965-1985) generations–were finally taken back to our mothers, and our mothers cared adequately for us, a deep first message of great uncertainties was imprinted, and even though we may bond, love, and have some happiness, we may never know with certainty that we can trust the love that we share. This could be one early primary explanation for why many of us, as adults, reach and seek for love and then when we get it, recoil in terror that this love is uncertain, and if we are to survive, we must remember that we are *bonded to separation*. This is a vicious cycle.

Given the impactful nature of the birth and bonding experience, it can indeed be difficult to alter those primary impressions, but it is not impossible. Much of my work with expectant couples is to help them recover for themselves the kind of fulfilling birth and bonding experiences they would desire to have if they could do it over. Then, through the actual births of their children, they can receive that experience for themselves as well. When parents strengthen their ability to make healthy choices for themselves, even in the face of past traumatic experiences, they are setting an example for their children in how to be powerful enough to make choices based on the present, rather than making their choices based on past traumatic or uncompleted experiences.

Imagine what it would be like if none of us had been separated from our mothers after birth at all. Would we possibly be able to develop our own sense of identity within a matrix of love and dependability rather than the need to be isolated? In traditional cultures, the norm has been to breastfeed and carry the children for two to four years.[9] This is not to say that this is the only way to have healthy bonding, but it is significant that this has been a cultural norm in so-called "primitive societies," which, in fact, demonstrate more wisdom about how to nurture children than we do[10], especially when we bond our children to technologies via plastic baby carriers instead of wraps and slings that keep our infants next to our bodies.

When we look at the United States since the 1940s, we can see that the major life transitions of birth and death have been removed from the home and brought into the hospital. The interdependent familial support systems for helping families through these significant transitions have been placed under the direction of hospital policy and procedures. The germ theory of disease, which gained ascendancy in the early 1900s, provided the justification for isolating newborns from their parents in hospital nurseries. Klaus and Kennell state, "As a result of problems of infection, maternity hospitals gathered full-term babies in large nurseries in a fortress-like arrangement. Germs were the enemy; therefore, parents and families who might carry them were excluded."[11] Most of the time, mothers in hospitals saw their newborn babies less than two hours a day. Klaus and Kennell go on to state,

> It often seems that practices based on 'expert opinion,' once established, are almost unchangeable, even though subsequent data and circumstances (such as the availability of antibiotics) make revisions appropriate. On the other hand, a practice such as keeping

a mother and baby together, which has been in existence for centuries, makes good common sense, ap-
peals to families, and is now supported by research
data, is extremely difficult to introduce and sustain in
a medical environment dominated by physicians' concerns about detecting and treating a variety of rare
conditions.[12]

Yet things have changed since then. Given that newborns often
got infections from being in nurseries full of other newborns and
of nurses who went from baby to baby, carrying contamination
with them, and the fact that bonding theory is now well-under-
stood, many hospitals have gotten rid of their nurseries in favor
of rooming-in, and that familiar picture of parents and relatives
staring at their babies through the nursery windows is slowly
becoming a thing of the past.

Frequently, mothers who do not see their babies for a long
time after the birth wonder if, when they do see their baby, it
is indeed theirs. In reporting on a summary of several studies,
Klaus and Kennell state,

What does seem apparent is that in a large number
of maternity units a mother in routine care who has
been totally separated from her child after a glimpse
at birth may not be sure the baby is healthy or even
breathing. She may not experience the flood of positive feelings that the beauty and responsiveness of her
baby could have released; she may feel lonely, empty,
deprived, and worried that the baby has some problem.[13]

I also know from my own work with families that many children with delayed maternal contact wonder if they were adopted and if their family is indeed their family. These kinds of feelings and concerns are evidence of uncompleted bonding experiences.

When babies are removed from their mothers immediately after birth, all of the physiological and hormonal mechanisms for bonding are occurring and the baby then bonds to whatever is available. This could be the feeling of isolation, a blanket, a whirring of a nearby motor, an incubator, a nurse, the sounds of other babies, etc. Many of us bonded primarily to objects or some form of technology, rather than bonding to human skin, touch, and love. This, for many of us of those generations, included bonding to a plastic nipple and bottle of milk rather than being breastfed, and being fed on a schedule rather than when we wanted to be fed.

Michel Odent has referred to a "cross-cultural negative attitude towards colostrum." Colostrum is the first liquid babies receive when they start nursing and continues until two or three days later when the milk comes in. Colostrum is high in antibodies for the baby, as well as certain essential proteins. It is scientifically proven to be the best substance newborns can receive in their first days. The fact that many cultures had, or have, taboos against breastfeeding a baby colostrum at birth does cause one to wonder about the deeper purpose behind such taboos. Dr. Odent believes that such taboos helped to ensure an aggressive attitude, and thereby helped one tribe be supreme over another. He states:

> Supremacy has lain with those who knew the cleverest ways to develop the human potential for aggression. One of the best ways to achieve this has been to disturb the first contact between mother and baby...It is no longer an evolutionary advantage to make humans

as aggressive as possible. The maxim should now be to maintain and cultivate a positive attitude to life. The priority is the genesis of an ecological human."[14]

If we accept Odent's premise, it may be no wonder why there is such a high level of violence and aggression in our society when we look at the birth and bonding practices that prevailed during the latter half of the 20th century.

It is important to know where we have come from as a society in our care and nurturing of newborns and their families, and it is also important to know where you, personally, have come from in your own experiences as a newborn and infant. What kind of an environment were you born into? Was your father or other parent present? Were you breastfed or bottle-fed? Was your mother excited and happy to see you? Or did she turn away from you? Did you have siblings to greet you? Knowing your own story of infancy can help you to prepare for parenting your newborn infant, and to provide the kind of environment in which you feel your baby will thrive.

Bonding involves the recognition of being wanted, loved, and accepted. Bonding after birth is the continuation of the process of bonding, which can occur prior to conception, at conception, and during pregnancy. Bonding involves all the five senses of touch, seeing, taste, smell, and hearing in an environment of pleasurable movement. Joseph Chilton Pearce has said, "Stillness is the enemy of the newborn." Yet stillness is precisely what we have given newborns after birth. It seems callous on our parts as a culture that we did not notice that the baby's intrauterine environment included continuous movement as well as sound, closeness to another physical being, and warm water. The environment of hospital nurseries does seem sterile and barren in comparison. Laura Huxley reports, "Recent research shows that lack of physical stimulation in the early months of life brings about a condition known as 'anedonia,' the inability to experience pleasure."[15]

What you are looking at in the bonding process as the mother or father is, "What does it take for me to lovingly and devotedly care for another, a developing human being?" The infant would be looking at the question, "What does it take for me to entrust myself into this person's care?" The infant gives the gift of receiving and the mother gives the gift of giving. When bonding is encouraged to happen in an uninhibited way, the process of connection and attachment occurs naturally. It is natural to love one another, to be close, to give and receive with another. It is natural to care for one another. In fact, it is in such an atmosphere of healthy dependency that the development of a strong self-identity can occur. When you feel deprived—either as a caregiver or care receiver—you may well have difficulty in feeling a strong sense of self-identity. Most of us learned that when we entrust ourselves to another, our needs are thwarted. As a parent, you can give your child a different experience of relationship—one in which needs are listened to and met, easily, in a context of fulfilling love. In doing so, you will be giving to yourself the kind of bonding experience that will help you complete your own infancy needs (Figure 4.2).

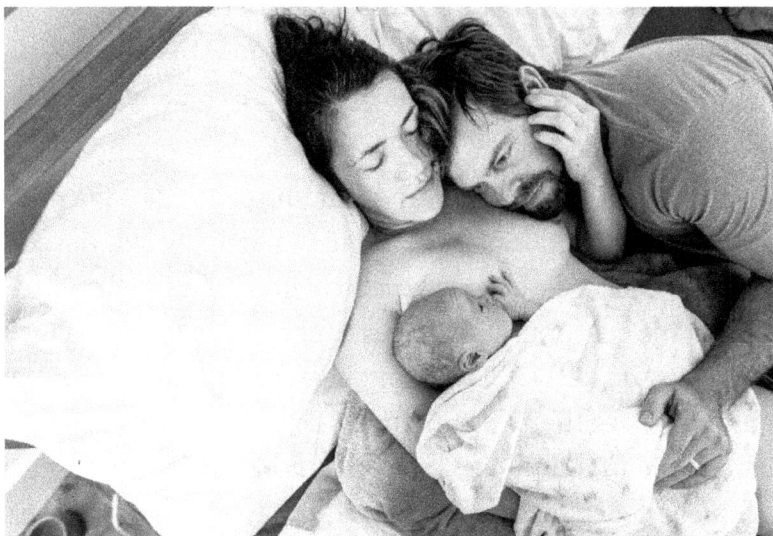

Figure 4.2. *This precious period after birth is often called "the Golden Hour." Photo by Monet Nicole, used with permission.*

WATER AND BONDING

Water can be a perfect matrix for the bonding process to occur. Water is a fluid, receptive environment, symbolizing the feminine. It is familiar, having been the baby's environment for nine months. Water is a conductor of energy and emotion, and allows for supported closeness and movement.

When you consider that the baby's environment for nine months has been water, you can see that placing the newborn in water after birth could be a comforting and familiar experience for him or her. Dr. Frederick Leboyer, a French obstetrician, wrote a book in the 1970s, *Birth Without Violence*. In it, he views birth from the baby's perspective, calling forth images of a gentle nature, soft lights, soothing, care-full touch, warmth, and relaxed caregivers. What he introduced that most captured the imagination of parents and caregivers alike was the placing of the baby in a warm bath soon after the birth. Hence, many parents began asking for the "Leboyer bath" for their newborn baby, which is a way of putting your baby in water soon after birth, even when she or he is not actually born in water.

Intuitively, many parents are drawn to warm water with their newborn. They seem to feel, if not know, that their infants like being in warm water. So even if they birth in a hospital, when they return home, they can frequently get into warm tubs with their newborns, as I often did. Infants often release stresses through movement, sound, and breathing while in the water and then go into a relaxed state of being, either alert and awake or asleep. Water also helps the parents to relax and go into a state of awareness that is more easily available to communications between them and their baby. Robbie Davis-Floyd, whose birth story appears in Chapter 2, provides an example of this type of communication in water:

> Once when my home-born son Jason was two, we were playing in the tub when it suddenly came to me to ask him what he remembered about his birth, about how he got born. He got a very fierce look on his face, starting making frog-like movements in the water, and said firmly, "I pushed with my head and I kicked with my feet!" I was blown away, and I suddenly understood that this birth had truly been a team effort. I had thought that I birthed him through my own efforts, but it turned out that he had been playing an active role too. I speculate that this is why he has always had a "can-do" attitude about life—his experience of birthing himself set up a positive pattern in his brain of "I can do this—whatever it is."

In addition to helping young children to remember their own births, being in water can help parents move from a "technological" orientation to parenting to an intuitive, inner knowing about parenting. From being with their babies in water, parents learn a great deal about themselves and their baby. Robbie also told me:

> When my kids were sick and too little to verbalize how they felt, I would always get in the tub with them, hold them close to my body, and ask them intuitively what was wrong. And I did not get out of the tub until I received an answer about what was wrong and what to do about it. Meanwhile my husband, who didn't believe in that sort of thing, would be calling our pediatrician to describe the child's symptoms. And to his astonishment, my answer and that of the doctor were always the same. I believe that being in water and holding your baby close facilitates intuitive connection and lets you hear what your child needs to tell you.

As Robbie describes, in the water, the parent can connect with their baby in ways that they, perhaps, may not be able to do on land. As a fluid, nonlinear medium, water enables the parent to be aware of the movements of the baby, of course keeping the baby's head above water, or helping the baby to move in the direction that he wishes to. Many babies and young children will want to dip their faces in the water, and parents learn to anticipate these dips and assist their child in going under and up in the water. Babies easily learn to hold their breath and seem to enjoy this form of play.

Dr. Odent states:

> The younger a baby is, the easier it is for him to swim. In the right environment, a baby can swim before he can walk. Of course, young human beings have an extraordinary capacity to learn, as long as it is in a joyful atmosphere...The human baby is perfectly adapted to water at birth. All he needs is the chance to cultivate this adaptation.

Odent goes on to report on the research of Igor Smirnov from St. Petersburg. Smirnov studied a group of children who swam regularly from birth on, and "came to the conclusion that the aquatic environment promotes early speech development."[16]

As mentioned in the preceding chapter, Igor Charkovsky of Russia has been researching and water training babies since the early 1960s and was still doing that until he died in 2021. He passionately believes in the benefits of early water training of infants. He believes that spending long stretches of time in warm water promotes brain development in the newborn because the water environment mitigates the effects of gravity on physiology. He feels that the energy babies expend in integrating the effects of gravity on their water-oriented systems does not allow them to develop parts of their brain that are able to develop in a weightless environment like water. He also feels that babies develop strong, well-coordinated bodies from their water training and claims that many have walked at age three months. He feels that anyone should be placed in water when they are ill and their body needs to heal, as easing the effects of gravity will allow the body to use that energy to heal itself. He has worked with over 10,000 children in various countries. Most of his views come from his own experience and intuitions and have not yet been studied in a scientific way. Nor has he published any papers about them, preferring to pass his methods on in person and via oral tradition. It is interesting to note, however, that his much-publicized work with infants has attracted thousands of people from all over the world to go to learn from him, so strong is the attraction to the use of water in birth and infancy.[17]

Michel Odent sees points of connections between the works of Dr. Leboyer and Charkovsky:

> In both cases there is water and there are newborn babies. Nobody knows better than Leboyer that, above all else, the newborn needs his mother's arms. But it was the artist Leboyer who gave the baby a bath. Interestingly enough, Leboyer introduced water into all his books and films. The work of Charkovsky has points in common with the work of Leboyer in so far as it is guided primarily by intuitions, faith, beliefs, feelings, clairvoyance; it is bound up with the unknown, mystery, perhaps even legend.[18]

Both of these men are known for their use of water in the birth and infancy experience. Since water is a symbol for the feminine, I can see that both of these men have symbolically been calling for the presence of the feminine as the safe and appropriate matrix for birth. It is important to also acknowledge the real, physical women who provide the oceanic environment for their baby's gestation, and birth their babies into the perfect matrix of their awaiting arms and energy fields. Women's inner knowing is the guiding force in a decision to use water at any point in the pregnancy, birth, and bonding process. Water can never replace an active, healthy, and consciously loving mother, but it is an environment that resonates harmoniously with the creative act of birth.

In birthing systems that have been dominated by the masculine approach to birth, it is difficult for many women to accept their own knowledge about the art of birth without also having the stamp of approval of male obstetricians. It takes courage for male obstetricians to come out publicly for the "feminine approach to birth." Dr. Odent, who has observed thousands of women giving birth, has acknowledged that he learned about birth from women themselves, not from textbooks or medical training. My feeling is that male obstetricians who are successful (peaceful, gentle, non-interventive) know that they are attending a birth in the service of the woman and her own unique birth dance, and not that the women are there to serve the obstetricians' model of how birth should be.

As women connect more and more with their own inner sources of power and trust their intuitions about birth[19], they will communicate to the established birthing system how they want to be assisted in their creative process of birthing. The two gifts I feel that obstetricians can give to women and birth are 1.) to give birth completely back to women; and 2.) to be sure that women have absolute privacy, protection, and security to uninhibitedly birth their babies just as they wish to.

This "call to water" that is appearing in the gentle and creative birth movement is, in a larger sense, a call to the remembrance of the perfection of the feminine—a feminine that is fertile, powerful, and fluid; a feminine that brings forth the fruit of her womb with graceful uninhibitedness; a feminine that is a bridge between Heaven and Earth; a feminine who is experiencing her own primal innocence in harmony and play with the masculine experiencing his innocence.

This "call to water" in birth is truly the Earth's baptism of her children into a more whole and harmonious relationship with all of the segments that combine to create a full and embodied human being. As I have noted in other chapters, when you consider that our children are arriving on a planet that is primarily water, you can see that it makes sense that the element of water be present as a ritual blessing of that individual's arrival.

I had a very real and impactful dream one night when I was in Hawaii. In the dream, I was a baby whale, inside my mother, about to be birthed. My grandmother was awaiting my arrival and to assist me to the surface for my first breath of air. I felt fear and did not want to come out but tried to hold onto the insides of my womb. My tail was coming out first. In the dream, another voice of mine asked, "Why would you not want to be birthed into this loving ocean and the presence of your family?"

The response of my baby whale self was, "Because I don't want to hear the human babies crying." My other self said, "Why are they crying?"

The response, "They are crying for water." Then I had a vision of these whale societies dedicated to "saving the human babies." I saw these whale societies throughout the oceans beaming their messages onto the earth to bring more of the fluidity of the ocean environment to birthing women and children, much as we have "Save the Whales" and "Save the Dolphins" movements.

After this dream, it occurred to me that perhaps the use of water in birth and infancy was not such an isolated, eclectic phenomenon meant for only a few. Perhaps there are millions of human babies desiring the blessings of water in their birth and infancy experiences. I do believe that babies and their families deserve to have the option and knowledge about the use of water in pregnancy, labor, delivery, and bonding readily available to them if they should choose to use them. This book has grown out of that belief.

In birthing and bonding with my children in water, I have always felt that the water was like liquid love, surrounding, caressing, and nurturing us, reminding me that I, too, was loved and supported in being a mother. If you could bathe yourself and your baby in this "liquid love," would that not be a pleasurable option to choose?

For those of you who say "yes" or "I'm interested," I offer the following possibilities to you. Please remember that these are not prescriptions for how to do it right, but possibilities to interweave in your own unique bonding process with your baby and your family.

WATER AND BONDING IN THE FIRST 24 HOURS

Perhaps you have labored and delivered your baby in warm water. If so, you will simply want to get yourself into a comfortable position so you can easily look at your baby and touch her. If you were in the squatting position, you may take an overturned pot or low stool with a foam pad on top to slip under your bottom. Your partner may already be sitting behind you, and you can relax back into their body. I have found that when my children were born, my first big desire was to look into their eyes. I would get myself into a position where I could easily see their eyes and was about twelve to eighteen inches from their faces. My oldest daughter Mela opened her eyes underwater and looked right at me. It was such a pleasure to have the closeness of our visual contact!

I have observed that the mother and the baby know when and how they desire to approach each other in various ways. Some are drawn to bring their baby up to their chest right away. Some like to look at each other for a long time, and perhaps the mother begins to touch or stroke the baby softly. When a baby comes out in the water—the same medium as in the womb—because they are not having to integrate the effects of gravity as much as if they were in the atmosphere, they are usually relaxed and able to pay close attention to their parents. Their body can be lifted, carried, or moved in gentle ways in the water without distracting them from the object of their focus, their mother (see Figures 4.3 and 4.4).

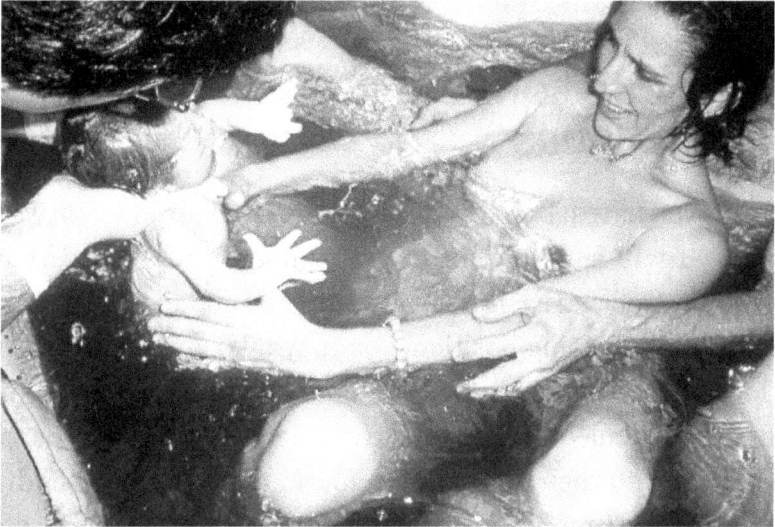

Figure 4.3. *Water birth in Brazil. Photo by obstetrician Adailton Salvatore, used with permission of the photographer and the mother.*

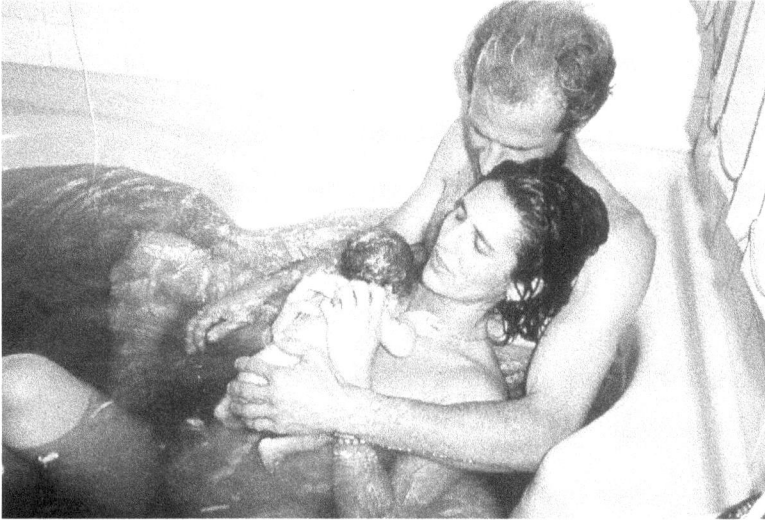

Figure 4.4. *Water bonding in Brazil. Photo by Adailton Salvatore, used with permission.*

I have usually stayed in the water with my newborns for twenty minutes to an hour after the delivery, simply because it was so comfortable and easy to be with them there. I wanted to have as little disturbance as possible from outside influences so we could revel in the joy and ecstasy of seeing and touching one another. It was also easy to float the baby into the crook of my arm and bring her close to my breast to suckle. I particularly liked introducing her to breastfeeding in this way because she was surrounded by warm water, except for her face, and I knew she was comfortable. It was easy for her to find the nipple and enjoy the first tastes of colostrum.

Babies and mothers are individuals. There is no one right way to proceed in bonding just after birth. Some babies want to suckle right away, some want a longer period of time of visual contact and holding, and some want to be gently stroked. When the baby starts making suckling motions, sticking their tongue in and out, they are ready to find the nipple. Most of them do perfectly well in finding and latching onto the nipple when they are placed next to the breast. You may assist them if you feel it is necessary by holding your breast steady or pressing your nipple up against the roof of their mouth. Breastfeeding shortly after birth facilitates the uterus in contracting, and if the placenta has not been delivered, nursing facilitates its delivery through the release of natural oxytocin.

For the (land) birth of her last baby, which her husband Uwe filmed, famed childbirth activist Sheila Kitzinger (now deceased), had the intuition not to touch her newborn immediately, nor to bring her up to the breast. Instead, she simply waited, and to her amazement, the baby crawled up her body and found the nipple on her own. This, too, can be achieved in the water; once babies swim up or are brought up to breathe, the water can facilitate their movements to find the breast on their own, as I have often observed.

Marshall and Phyllis Klaus have identified seven states of consciousness in the newborn infant: quiet sleep, active sleep, drowsiness, quiet alert, active alert, and crying.[20] At birth, the "traditional" crying of the baby is not necessarily so traditional. Parents who have birthed their babies in gentle ways with a minimum of interventions have seen that their babies most likely arrive in the quiet alert stage. Some parents have expressed worry that their babies did not cry at birth. Yet, *crying is not mandatory for showing that the baby is healthy.* When babies cry at birth, it is usually because they are releasing some stress from the birth experience. If this occurs with your baby, simply allow your baby to cry and let him know that you are listening to him. You may have a strong intuition about just what he is expressing. Maybe his head hurts, or a certain part of his body is uncomfortable. Whatever it is, the best thing to do is not to try and stop the crying, but to receive the crying as the expression he needs to make in order to relieve whatever stress he is experiencing. Sometimes, I have heard babies cry at birth and have felt that it was a part of a final grieving process about leaving the womb and accepting the expanded extra-uterine environment.

The art of conscious communication (communion) is what bonding is all about. During the first twenty-four hours, you are in a special love nest with your newborn. Every system of the newborn—physiological, emotional, mental, and spiritual—is opened and flowing towards you as a mother, and each of your systems are opened and flowing towards your baby. If you had an unmedicated birth, the channels for communication and awareness are open and heightened by your hormonal system. You literally experience the separation of your baby's body from your own and see his own special uniqueness, while at the same time being in a context of union and love. If there is one state of consciousness I could recommend to enhance the bonding process, particularly in this first twenty-four hours, it would be the state of consciousness that sees no conflict between simultaneous individuation and unification. Some people call this unconditional acceptance and love. Often, people learn about this state of consciousness from the birthing and bonding process itself, and have such profound experiences that they feel their lives are altered in a positive way from that time on.

Another key state of consciousness that nourishes this first twenty-four hours is a consciousness that lets the baby know that they do not have to leave behind or forget anything they considered valuable in the world they came from prior to conception—the non-physical realm, and the world of the physical they have come into. In other words, you are acknowledging the existence of life beyond that which we perceive with our physical senses—the place where babies come from. Wouldn't you feel strange if you moved from the United States to Russia and the people there didn't want you to tell them anything about the United States or acknowledge you came from a different place at all? That is similar to how you may view the changes a baby is making in coming from one realm of existence to another. To have a consciousness that is open to a newborn's previous experience, whatever that may be, is a wonderful gift. I believe such a state of consciousness will allow babies to bring with them valuable knowledge, skills and abilities that can help them and others in the physical world. You will then be giving your baby a message of acceptance about the totality and depth of their existence and experience. Such an acceptance can give them a foundation for being incredibly vibrant and alive human beings.

Transitions are the ways we move from one place to another to weave the past with the present and the present into the future. What you do and how you are with your newborn is consequential in establishing their reality of life (as well as yours). I believe that you and your baby have come together because your unique responses to each other are appropriate for one another. I have heard many parents say that they feel their baby is their teacher. This reflects to me that there is reciprocal learning if you are open to that kind of relationship with your child. Another example of this kind of communication from baby to parent is when parents who would never have known about or considered using water in their birthing experience suddenly find they are dreaming about water and being with their baby in water. Then they read a newspaper article or see a video about water birth and find themselves asking, "I wonder if we could find a place where we could use water in our birth?" Parents tell me that many times they feel guided by their baby in bringing together all the elements they desire in their birthing experience.

In the first hours after birth, by open-heartedly revealing yourself to your baby, you are providing them with a multifaceted and multidimensional picture of reality—a picture that they imprint into their physiology, emotions, minds, and spirits. First impressions tend to register deeply. Newborns' impressions at this catalyzing point of birth will be impressions they will use to learn about and understand their reality from then on. As human beings, I feel it is natural for us to want to make good impressions, and certainly at birth, this desire is present with most parents. You want the best for your baby. You want your baby to feel that life is worth living, that there is meaning, beauty, truth, and joy in this physical reality, and that pain or obstacles or discomforts can be moved through in safe and beneficial ways.

There is so much richness and opportunity in bonding with your newborn—so much to feel, hear, see, smell, know, and do. The element of water adds to your bonding experience a medium that lets your creativity flow, as well as your baby's.

If you delivered your baby outside of a tub, you may find that you feel like holding your baby and stepping into a tub to relax and bond, or you may not feel like entering the water together until much later. Sometimes, parents and babies bond and nurse for a while, and then either enter a tub or bring over a baby bath of warm water, the "Leboyer bath." You can easily hold your baby in the warm water and continue your face-to-face communication. Often upon entering a warm bath, babies immediately relax and sometimes smile. Sometimes, babies will grimace and cry, allowing the warm bath to help them release some emotions from the birth. Afterwards, these babies go into a relaxed alert state. Babies also fall asleep quite easily in a warm bath (with someone holding their head up, of course), showing us how comfortable the water is to them. I can see how waterbed bassinets for babies could feel quite good to them.

Being with the baby in a large or small bath is also a wonderful way for the father to connect and bond with the baby. In my three water bonding experiences, I left the tub to dry off and get comfortable in my bed while my husband floated the babies and bonded with them in the tub. It was a special, quiet time for him to share with them. When they left the tub and were brought to me, they nursed and fell into a deep, peaceful sleep.

During this first twenty-four-hour period, I felt intuitively that each of my babies wanted to be in the water two or three times. I or my husband would play in the tub with them for up to an hour, keeping the water a constant warm temperature by adding warm water. They seemed to enjoy the sound of the water trickling into the tub. Sometimes, I would float my babies with one hand behind their necks as they slept in the water. The message I wanted to impart to them was that the pleasures of the womb were still available to them along with the new pleasures of being outside the womb.

When babies are in a quiet alert phase in the water, they will stretch their fingers, arms, and legs, turn their heads, and learn about the movements of their body without running into the walls of the womb as they did prior to birth. Sometimes, I would hold them so their feet would push into my abdomen, giving them the experience of pushing off with their legs and then going on a little floating trip around the tub. These movements are, of course, done on land as well. However, in the water, babies can do these movements in a much more circular, fluid, and supported way.

On the first day, I also experimented with playing familiar music to the baby during bath time. I had picked three tapes of music that I played during my pregnancy, at times during labor, and then again after the birth. I found that one of the tapes, which was meditative and slow, would soothe my babies and put them into a deep sleep in the bath.

A key to bonding during this first day is privacy—a great deal of privacy for the mother, baby, and nuclear family. I suggest that close family or friends who do come to greet the baby should come after the first half of the day and, of course, blend in with the atmosphere and the energy of the baby. Remember, this is your baby's first twenty-four hours outside the womb. Allow your baby to be the guiding influence in the activities and greetings of the day.

WATER AND BONDING: THE FIRST WEEK

During the next six days, your baby will be learning a great deal about herself and her body, adapting to life outside the womb. She will learn about suckling, digestion, excretion, breathing, movement, touching and being touched, hearing, seeing, smelling, and tasting, about being hungry and being full, and about communicating her needs to you. As parents spend time getting to know their baby, they gradually learn to put themselves in their infant's place. When they do, the signals the baby sends out to make his or her needs known or to elicit a response become increasingly clear. Within us all are amazing inborn systems for communicating, nurturing, and surviving.[21] Your baby will also be learning a great deal about you and her family. Her interactive and communicative life increases tremendously. Childrens' brains up to age 2 develop more neural networks faster than at any other time in their lives, and those neural networks get formed in response to whatever environment they find themselves in. So as parents, we need to do our best to ensure that those environments are beneficial, loving, and stimulating.

When I talk about privacy during early bonding, I don't mean a privacy in which nothing is happening, but rather a privacy that honors the wealth of experience occurring within and between the parents and their baby. Being with your baby during the first week is really a time of tuning into her and yourself and working out a harmonious relationship. I have found it impossible to live my life with a new baby based on preconceived pictures of what I think should occur. For first-time parents, this can be frustrating. Often, what used to be priority projects are now way down on the list, such as housecleaning and organizing, not to mention eight hours of straight sleep. As parents, we learn to trust a new wisdom and flow about living our lives as caretakers of a new and developing human being. That is why the choice to have a baby is so important. The job is not over once the baby is here. It is a joyous job, and one that can profoundly alter you forever. That, to me, is why we have the particular children we have, because they come to bring us gifts of learning, just as we give to them.

During this first week, your baby will be teaching you things about yourself, if you allow that by choosing to adopt the perspective that you are also learning from your baby. One of the first things you may learn about yourself with your newborn is more about how you felt as a newborn with your parents. Particularly, if you were not breastfed, you may find yourself having feelings of resentment for no apparent reason. If you look carefully and deeply, you may find that there is an infant within you who has feelings that want to be expressed. If you give that infant within you permission to feel those feelings, you will be giving yourself the great gift of nurturing and developing the full human being that you are. As you parent your newborn, you will also be parenting the infant within you. As you listen to and accept your infant's feelings, you will be integrating uncompleted aspects of yourself and finding a freer and happier you.

To realize that your baby does not cause you to have any frustrations you may experience, but rather allows you to see frustrations already within you, is a healthy attitude to adopt when learning to parent a newborn. If you have previously learned something about how to parent yourself, you will be starting your parenting of your newborn from a firm foundation.

You can really have a fun and creative time giving to your infant the kinds of love, communication, and pleasure that you would like to be giving yourself. What would feel good to you if you were a newborn? What would you like to see, hear, feel, and do? Who would you like to spend time with? Being able to answer these questions for yourself will certainly help you to tune into your baby, his feelings, and his desires.

Breastfeeding, with the full honest-to-goddess milk flowing in on the second or third day, is certainly the highlight of the first week. Babies look absolutely satiated, happy, and high when full of the nourishment of their first meal of breastmilk. Until supply and demand work themselves out in a more equitable fashion, there is usually an abundance of milk, definitely more than the baby needs to feel full. When looking at my child's happy face sleeping under a breast still dripping milk along her cheek, I felt that breastfeeding is an impactful experience of *bonding with the reality of abundance*. I have wondered whether, if we had all bonded with the experience of an abundance of breastmilk always there just when we wanted it, we would not have the problems with supply and demand of all forms of nourishment being in the right place at the right time that we have in our contemporary world. If we all had experienced an abundance of breastmilk as babies, would we feel more abundant in our lives as adults? I believe we would.

Many mothers have told me how much they enjoy breast-feeding their babies in a warm bath. Certainly, it allows the mother to be more uninhibited, since she can let the excess milk drip in the tub and doesn't have to deal with pads, rags, or milk running down her body. I recommend filling the tub as full as you can so that you can either sit up comfortably and cradle your baby in your arms, or lean back, perhaps against an inflatable pillow, and nurse semi-reclining. You and your baby will learn the positions and ways that feel most comfortable to you both. I found breastfeeding in a bath to be relaxing for me, as well as for my babies. I also feel that it helped them in digesting the milk.

In the Soviet Union, Igor Charkovsky, as part of his water training activities, suggested that mothers lower their babies underwater for a brief second or two while feeding and then bring them back to the surface. He felt this would help the babies be comfortable with putting their faces underwater and holding their breath. He said that when they are sucking, they are holding their breath and can easily go under and up, and that doing this two or three times a feeding can be helpful in developing their water abilities. However, I recommend doing this only if it feels joyful, playful, and intuitively appropriate for your baby and you. I will write more about water training and baby swimming in the next section.

Another activity that can be enjoyable to introduce in the first week is massaging your baby. Certainly, it can be done out of the water, and it is also fun to do massage in the water. Simply lean back in the tub with your knees up and lay your baby face up on your thighs. Usually, you can raise or lower your knees to get more or less water flowing over your baby's body. In this position, it is easy to begin with the feet and use stroking, kneading, and circular motions all over the foot and toes and up each leg. (There are some excellent infant massage books available if you would like help in developing your techniques. One of them is *Infant Massage* by Vimala Schneider McLure.) Once you complete the legs, go to the hands and arms, and repeat the same process. Allow yourself to move with your baby's movement of his arms or legs. Then, you can move to the torso and use long sweeping motions from the top of the chest down onto the abdomen, and use clockwise circular motions on the abdomen. You will be able to alter your massage according to your baby's responses to you. You can tell if your baby is open and receptive to your strokes, or if your baby is preferring to do something else. Usually, they are open and receptive. At some point during the massage, they may cry. If they cry and are still open and receptive, simply know they are releasing emotional energy and let them know you are listening and receiving what they have to say. When the emotion passes, they will usually be calm and happy. If they cry and pull away, discontinue the massage to let them know you are listening to their communication. You can continue the massage when you feel they are open and available to it once again. You can gently massage their face and scalp with small circular motions. They quickly develop strong cheek muscles from their suckling, and I imagine that massaging their cheeks and foreheads would feel good to them, just as it does to us.

To massage their back, simply lean back in the tub yourself and lay your baby face down on your chest. From this position, you can use kneading, squeezing, and circular strokes along their back and buttocks. You can also gently rub the back of their head and neck. Throughout all the massage, you can keep warm water flowing over their body either with your hands or by raising or lowering your legs. Baby massage—in water or on a bed—is also another great way for fathers/partners to bond and participate with their baby in a sensitive and caring way.

WATER AND BONDING: THE FIRST THREE MONTHS

As you and your baby grow more and more familiar with each other, feeling safe, secure, and competent, you may want to introduce your baby to more activities both in and out of the water. From living in the womb, your baby is already adapted to water, having a "diving reflex." This reflex automatically closes the baby's air passages when underwater to keep the baby from inhaling water. Since this reflex is active until around six months of age, introducing baby swimming activities can be a way to keep this reflex alive without your infant having to relearn to hold her breath at a later time. Most baby swim classes start at age three months. However, if you feel confident about swim activities with your baby, you can begin them any time after birth. Also, at around three months of age, the bathtub is getting a little small for baby swimming, so going to a larger pool with other mothers and babies can be the next step in interesting water activities for your child.

To begin water swimming, hold your baby's face toward the water with one hand under each armpit. You can move the baby through the water this way. When you get ready to dip her under, look directly into her eyes, smile, take a deep breath, and blow into her face, immediately and gently dipping her under and up in the water. Make some positive acknowledgement to her and continue with another more familiar and comforting water movement. Your baby will automatically hold her breath when you blow in her face, and this becomes a signal that she will be going underwater. Eventually, you will not even need to blow in her face; she will simply sense it intuitively from your voice or actions. I found that dipping my babies three to six times a swim was usually enough to be integrated into the whole swim session. Occasionally, your baby may accidentally swallow some water. Hold her face down out of the water and allow her to cough or splutter until the water is cleared. Then, hold her and soothe her until she is calm. The calmer and quieter the environment is, and the calmer you are, the less these occasional mishaps will occur.

I have discovered that when mothers or fathers feel joyful and safe about swimming activities with their infant, the baby feels joyful and safe. Charkovsky has said that babies usually have no fear of the water on their own, but rather learn to fear water from their parent's fear. Many adults have a fear of water, which could stem from their own birth experience if their umbilical cord was cut too soon and they choked on amniotic fluids. Many of us had traumatic experiences when we learned to swim and felt forced to go underwater. It is wise to share about your water experiences as an infant or child with your partner as a way to release any fears or negative experiences you have had.

If water is safe and fun for you, chances are that it will certainly be safe and fun for your infant. I would not recommend water training activities with your baby if you do not feel comfortable in the water yourself. Obviously, you should never leave your baby alone in or around water. I would also not recommend water training activities if your baby definitely shows you he does not want to learn baby swimming or do any other water activity. Of course, if your baby has any ear problems, I would not recommend swimming underwater until they are cleared up. Otherwise, water is a safe and therapeutic medium for your infant.

During these first three months, your baby and you will be continuing to grow and learn about one another. This new relationship takes time and attention, which means that you, as a mother, need to have support, just as your newborn has your support. This is no time to be the supermom who does everything herself *and* cares for her newborn. Traditionally, we've had larger extended families living in close proximity to one another, and grandmothers, aunts, and older siblings helped out with day-to-day activities so the new mother and new baby could focus on one another. We rarely have those today. Getting the rest and nourishment you need means living in harmony with your baby's rhythms. I have experienced that receiving a good therapeutic massage at least once a week in the first three months is beneficial for the new mom. Your body is reorganizing to breastfeeding and carrying your infant on the outside, and your uterus and pelvic muscles are re-adapting to their pre-pregnant state. Taking walks with your baby, doing gentle yoga, and new mother stretches are also beneficial.

Be sure you take some time for yourself, even if it's only twenty minutes to take a shower, nap, or short walk on your own. Ask your partner or friends to be with the baby for brief periods while you do some relaxing activity for yourself. If you have a new mothers' support group in your area, I recommend attending. Such groups are a wonderful way to share with other understanding mothers and babies. Also, there may be infant massage classes available for both mothers and fathers. All of these activities will help you, your partner, and any other children, in your transition to becoming the new expanded family that you are.

There may be times when it feels appropriate to share the bath time with older siblings. My older girls loved to watch my son, Hank, at his bath time. Even though they were not in the water with him, they would sit by the tub and applaud and acknowledge him every time he did one of his unique water activities. When we graduated from the bathtub into a larger hot tub, the whole family could participate. Since my two girls both had early water training, it was not long before we all felt confident in allowing them brief periods of holding Hank and playing with him in the water. Also, in the larger hot tub, I would "play baby" with my older girls and do some of the activities with them that I did with Hank. They loved it and it helped them to feel as special and cared for as the newborn.

Occasionally, in these first three months, babies will go through fretful periods, sometimes known as colic. These can be brief or prolonged, mild or intense. Frequently, they occur around the same time each day for a while, usually in the evening. If this occurs with your infant, consult with your midwife or pediatrician. Often, colic is related to digestive disturbances and many times, it is emotional. I had one child with regular crying periods for several weeks and discovered that it seemed to be one thing on one day and another the next. There is a particular kind of acidophilus made for infants that helps them with digestion, which you can find at most Whole Foods and other stores. Warm water and infant massage are also soothing and calming both for their digestive tract and emotions. If your infant has longer spells of crying, be sure you have support so that you can let others be with the baby as well. The best thing you can do is to go off and take time to release your stress so that you can continue to give a receptive and calm environment to your baby. Often, listening to your baby, tuning in to what he is trying to communicate, and verbally talking to him about whatever it is you feel is going on with him can also help a great deal.

BENEFITS OF WATER AND BONDING

- Water provides a familiar medium for the baby so the baby has fewer new inputs to integrate at one time and can thus focus on bonding.
- Water allows for gentle movement of the baby into the mother's arms after delivery, without needing to move his body in gravity.
- Water is warm and keeps the baby from any sudden temperature changes.
- Remaining in a warm bath after a birth allows the mother to not have to move to a different location and to be kept warm herself. It can also help to ease the pain of afterbirth contractions.
- Sitting in the warm bath with her newborn allows the mother to be comfortable, to relax, and to have privacy from interruptions.
- Being in warm water for the first breastfeeding allows maximum skin-to-skin contact without the need for blankets or caps.
- Returning a newborn to a warm bath after birth is a reminder that the pleasures of the womb are available outside of the womb, and assists the baby in making an easy transition to a new gravity-based environment.
- Water is buoyant and assists the baby in moving easily, as

well as in making movements that would be more difficult out of the water.

- ♦ Water provides a comfortable and safe medium in which fathers or partners can hold and move their babies and have special fun time with them.

- ♦ Water is a great fitness activity for the infant, allowing for optimal muscle development, coordination, and balance, which then transfer to his ability to move on land.

- ♦ Since babies are used to being in movement in the womb, water bonding continues the familiarity of gentle movement.

- ♦ Movement in water stimulates brain development and right and left hemisphere coordination.

- ♦ Water activity continues the baby's adaptation to water begun in the womb, building on the great amount of growth and learning that occurred during pregnancy.

- ♦ Teaching the baby to hold her breath underwater and float in water helps her to be water-safe as she grows up.

- ♦ Water bonding helps parents to relax and feel comfortable playing with their infants, perhaps reminding the parents of fun water play when they were children.

- ♦ Water can help babies to relax when they are fretful or have colic.

- ♦ Water can aid the digestive process in the infant and the milk let-down reflex of the mother.

- ♦ Water conducts energy and emotion from mother to baby, aiding in their communication process.

RISKS OF WATER AND BONDING: HOW TO AVOID THEM

- ◊ Never put or keep a baby in water who does not indicate receptivity and openness to being in the water.

- ◊ If you are afraid and worried about water bonding activities, your baby will most likely exhibit fear and anxiety also.

- ◊ Do not initiate water bonding with your baby when you are feeling stressed or distracted from calm and full attention on your baby.

- ◊ Do not do water bonding with your baby from preconceived "shoulds" about water, but simply as pleasurable and relaxing time with your baby.

- ◊ If you are not fully attentive to your baby, there is a risk that the baby will swallow water, sputter, and choke.

- ◊ Never leave your baby alone in or near water, or in the care of a sibling or adult who is afraid of the water.

- ◊ Be careful that the water temperature is just right, body temperature, not too cool or too warm, and that it is not overly chemicalized and uncomfortable to your baby's eyes or skin.

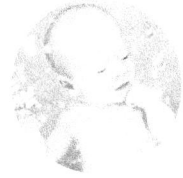

PERSONAL STORIES ABOUT WATER, PREGNANCY, AND BIRTH

Personal Account: Water and Bonding

Maria and Wayne Mathias, and Julian Mathias, Moline, Illinois.

Wayne: The most impactful water experience I had with Julian was the birth itself and being with him for at least thirty minutes while Maria was being attended to beside the birthing tub. I was so high during the whole thing that to relate that now in normal consciousness is difficult. What I did with him was to hold him in what we call "handling places" so he could participate and move in the water. Handling places are places on the body that allow him to move and not be penned in. An example is just behind the chest so he could move in a multidirectional way. I was trying to make it comfortable for him to mobilize his body in the water. When we first pulled him out of the water and gravity took his body, he went totally limp, like a marshmallow melting into your hands. When he was back in the water, he was strong enough with the aid of the water to move around. I cradled him with a hand under his upper and lower back. He could move his legs and arms and squirm his body. I didn't want to impede his movements at all. He was rather weak at first, but then his movements got stronger.

In bonding with him, I was aware that here was a new little entity, and I knew he was not me. I was amazed that this whole little human being had come from Maria and me. I was fully focused on him and was drawn to be delicate and supportive.

He and I were practically inseparable from that moment on. The bonding that happened was that I focused on him that first thirty minutes and it's never stopped since then. I became fully aware of him being a part of my life from that time on. At the beginning, bonding wasn't much of a two-way street because he was kind of in a free fall, still coming into his experience. He opened his eyes, squinted underwater, and looked at both of us before we brought him up. It felt like that was his intention, to roll over and look at each of us. It was like he was saying, "Look, I've been listening to these voices for so long. Who is this?"

Maria: I was still in the birth process and pretty out of it at the time Julian came out. I felt relieved that he was out and was okay. It took me pretty much all day to realize that I had a baby. I remember that night I realized I wasn't pregnant anymore. After the delivery, I was ready to get out of the water. I didn't nurse him until he was lying down by me on the bed. We looked into each other's eyes, and he was real, real aware. This was after he was in the tub with Wayne. That was just about the coolest thing to me. I made a deep connection with him at that time. It was perfect that Wayne and Jules had such an important time together. Wayne was in total, total ecstasy. I don't think I've ever seen him so happy!

Wayne: In the water, I recall kind of soothing him, even singing, I think. I was totally engaged with him. We had our own little energetic womb. There were telephone calls and people moving around, and I remember feeling that those were incredible intrusions into our little world in the tub. The whole ambiance of being together with him that first 30 minutes was so delicate that anyone getting close to it felt like having cold water thrown on me. I think I was partially in shock because he was a boy. Early on, I had a deep feeling he was a boy. It was obvious to me then. Later on in the pregnancy, Maria said she felt like the baby was a female. For some reason, I gave up the knowing I had. I just gave up thinking I could be so lucky to have a boy. When he came out, I was astounded. I had already spent 10 years with our little girl—her showing me the world and me showing her the world. I knew it would be a different experience to have a little boy, who would bring up all my childhood experiences. Now, we have two boys and two girls in this house. It's a different situation. I didn't even think in those terms prior to his birth, of what it would mean to me to have him be a boy. It made it even more incredible to me. I hadn't even considered that I would be raising a boy. After his birth, I felt graced to have a boy because I already had a girl. I was pretty much in an altered state for a week or more.

Water has always been a big part of his experience. The first week, we would spend up to an hour in the tub. It gave him the ability to have some control over his movement, skin-to-skin contact, and real soothing. From the first week on, you could tell his deep love for water. Now, if he even sees water or hears the sound of water, his face lights up. He just took to it right away. He loved floating on his back and kicking. The water was a big deal for me. It was one of the ways I could feel like I was communicating with him. He did a lot of screaming, chortling, and splashing, which he didn't do much outside of the water. He was able to express joy in the water more than out of the water. One of the comments we had about Julian was that he enjoys being alive. He enjoys being alive more than anyone we've ever met. That joy was expressed more in the water than anywhere else. He would carry on and have a great time.

Maria: At about six weeks, we took him to the pool. We thought, maybe, it would be too cool, but he loved it. I tried nursing him and dipping him under the water once and didn't feel comfortable in doing that process. I knew from Igor's work that if the parent is scared, that fear can be passed on to the baby. I didn't want to do underwater swimming until I felt more confident myself.

Wayne: I did blow in his face and dip him a few times. He did swallow some water. I tried to weigh the value; is it worth it to try and break through this and possibly lose his trust? I didn't want him to not trust me, so I was cautious about dipping him.

Maria: I always felt like he would like to do more swimming underwater, but we were not prepared. I just didn't have the courage to be as confident and relaxed about baby swimming as I think I could have been. We took him to baby swim classes when he was six months old. Jules would be in the water as long as you would be in the water. He would even take little naps in there, especially after nursing in the warm bath.

One thing I observed about Jules being in the water a lot every day was that it would make him stronger and more energetic, and I think he needed to sleep less outside of the water. Sometimes, I don't think that was always a benefit to me when I would be ready for him to go to sleep. His waking periods would be longer after his water experiences. I do believe the water strengthened his constitution. We always measured his progress by the way he was in the water.

Wayne: I'd like to tell other fathers who might be wanting to do water bonding with their newborn that the important thing for me with Julian is that I'm just hanging out and being with him in the water. I'm not really *doing* anything. I know for a lot of men that it's real hard to hang out and not do anything. If a man gets in the tub with his baby to wash him, it's "do this, do that." I don't think it would have the same kind of chemistry as what I'm talking about with Jules. Being in the water with Julian is definitely my highlight time with him. Maria has other highlight times with him, and the water time is my special time with him. I think fathers don't feel like they really get to do things with their baby until the baby is many months old. I feel that the water bonding activities provide an opportunity for those fathers that want to have a special time with their newborn. I recommend to fathers who want to do this to support spontaneous behavior in the water and let go of agendas. After you do it a few times, you get the idea and it's fun. I think the message or feeling you impart to your baby when you do this is that there's a lot of support available for the baby—unconditional support. The child has the experience of being able to be independent and supported at the same time. The water is supporting the independent movement and the father is supporting the baby. I think the message that comes across to the baby is that "I can move from my own center and still be supported." Jules and I do a lot of communicating with one another. I talk or sing to him, and he listens. I feel like I am able to be with him at his level and it's so rewarding! Another thing I like about being in the tub with him is that there are no distractions. I can't be anywhere else in the house without some form of distraction likely to occur. In the tub, it's just me and him, hanging out. He's doing his silly stuff and so am I.

Maria: I'm glad water is in Jules' life. I think it is a positive linkage to his birth experience and makes me think that his birth experience was positive for him. I don't know why Wayne has responded to him with such strong bonding as he has. I don't know if this would have occurred so easily for him out of the water as it did in the water. In the water, he was able to take over a central role while I was feeling like getting out of the water. My water work was over, and Wayne's was beginning. We didn't have it planned this way, but now, I see the perfection in how it did occur and the miracle of the wonderful relationship they have. Wayne's behavior in other ways is more like a mother would be. For example, if Jules is crying in the night, Wayne is just as likely as me to be up out of bed in a second to pick him up. With Aria, he was definitely attentive and loving, but not to the point of being keyed in just like a mother would be. With Jules, Wayne took on the role of the father right away. It took me a progression of days, probably weeks, to fully bond and be the mother. My bonding with Aria seemed to be more instantaneous, more like Wayne's with Jules. I didn't realize that there would be these kind of differences for us in bonding with a boy instead of a girl. Both of our children are wonderful, and they both have their own unique energies. I'm grateful we learned about water birth and water bonding for Jules' birth.

Personal Account:
Water and Bonding—Birth Attendant

by Barbara Harper, Santa Barbara, California

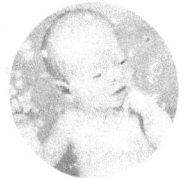

I've attended hundreds of water births. One of the things I've observed with women who have birthed in the water is that they have so much available energy and attention as soon as the baby's out. Their focus is in the present. In births I've attended in other places, either hospital or home, without the use of a tub, the attention tends to be more easily distracted. Water seems to intensify the parent's ability to concentrate on the baby. In every water birth that I've observed so far, the women have all breast-fed their babies while they are still in the water. They leave the baby half submerged, cradled in the crook of the elbow.

In my own experience as a mother, I didn't want to leave the bath when the baby was born. I hadn't necessarily planned to stay in the tub after the birth. I just found that I didn't want to get out. I loved being there. We had a wonderful jacuzzi outdoors by the bedroom and it was lovely there, a warm November day. With Abraham, I stayed in the water almost 2½ hours. I delivered the placenta there, breastfed him there, and when I got sleepy, I was ready to get out. The baby even slept in the water. His father held him and played with him in the water also. I don't think I would have had the same availability of my energy if I hadn't been in the warm water, because the after-birth contractions were pretty painful. I don't know if I could have been as comfortable and present for my baby with that pain outside of the tub. Those contractions were more painful than the labor contractions. In the tub, I was able to have a wonderful experience bonding with my baby because the pain was minimized by the water.

I've observed that fathers get in the tub with their baby and don't wait for someone to hand them the baby or give them permission to touch their baby. They reach down and seem to naturally want to hold and be with their baby. Water seems to bring the whole family unit closer together. It seems easier to be close physically, as well as emotionally. Frequently, the father stays in the tub while the mother gets out, cleans up, and lies down on the bed. Seeing the father with the baby in the tub is almost like seeing another mother with the baby, so attentive and complete is their connection. I've seen attentive fathers outside of the water too, but all the fathers that I've watched in the tub were totally engrossed. Dads don't want to relinquish that time. It is so special to them. Most fathers get back into the tub the next day with their newborn. I've seen a number of fathers take it upon themselves to run a bath and once again, have that close, special time with their baby.

I've also watched a lot of children get into the water with their new sibling. They have been standing there wide-eyed, the tub has been set up for a week, and they want to immediately take their clothes off and get in. I remember a 3-year-old who had slept through the birth. We went in and woke him up, and the minute he saw his baby brother, he was ready to take his clothes off and get into the tub. The new family unit stayed in the water for a good half hour. Everyone else stayed out of the room and were respectful and quiet. People seem to enjoy the sensual warmth of the water. You have said before, Rima, that the water is like liquid love, and that's what I always see when I look at a family like that. The whole family is encased in liquid love.

The first week or two after birth, I've seen a lot of moms and dads do relaxation exercises with the baby in the water. They'll float the baby with one hand under the back of the head, gently gliding the baby through the water. The other thing they do is support the baby under their arms and their chin, and glide them that way. Frequently, the babies do a kicking motion when they are gliding through the tub. These parents seem happy to be able to provide their babies with such a flexibility in being able to move by having them in the water. They have also been amazed at how readily a fussy baby will quiet down in the water. I always recommend trying a warm water bath for a fussy baby.

One of the things that a baby in the water will teach an adult is that if there's any tension in your body, the baby will pick up on it. When you're floating a baby, you have to surrender to that baby and consciously go through your body and see where you're holding tension. One woman said to me, "I was in the jacuzzi with the baby, and she was really fussing. I realized that my shoulders were really tight. When I let go of my tightness, the baby really calmed down." Babies reflect back to us where we have problems. That's magnified in the water. The baby just won't let you "pass" unless you relax too. Dads have also told me the same thing. Being in the tub with your baby is a time that you have to be totally present for them. You can't be thinking about something else. They know when you're not present for them, and their reaction will jerk you back into the present.

Some parents, including myself, continue water swimming with their babies, teaching them to hold their breath and go underwater. I used the book by Virginia Hunt Newman on baby swimming. It's "one, two, three, blow in their face, and put them under." I did that with my son and have watched several other couples do the same. We all found it a wonderful time to enjoy being with our newborns. One couple's little one-month-old was swimming underwater and enjoying it. Now she's a year and a half and she just can't wait to jump in the water. I haven't seen any problems with swallowing water and choking. It seems to be our fear and not theirs. I've also watched babies who love to mimic their parents. They will put their face in the water if you do, or they will blow bubbles if you blow bubbles. Your enjoy-ment of the water teaches your baby to enjoy the water.

I have seen one baby who loves her bath time but neither of the couple swims. The baby cries when you take her out of the bath. I think she would have liked to spend more time in the water if her parents had been willing to take her in more often. Parents need to listen in to their babies and feel what it is they want. Some babies just have a love of water. I recommend for parents to get over any fears they have of water (using the methods Rima recommends in Chapter 1) so they can feel confi-dent with a baby who wants to be in the water.

I think birth attendants should encourage parents to continue water bonding activities with their baby after birth. Especially for a first-time mom, there is a relaxation that can be achieved in the water after the birth that might not be as easy on land. Prenatal classes should definitely include postpartum water bonding activities. Sometimes, midwives will put women in the bath either to deliver the placenta, clean up, or to bond with the baby. So, even if a couple hasn't had a water birth, they should have the option to get in the water with their baby after birth, for relaxation, easing pain, and bonding. I also think attendants need to be careful to look at their own fears about actually seeing a baby come out underwater so that if a woman is instinctively drawn to water, the birth attendant will not be putting his or her judgements on the use of water but will feel as safe and confident as in a birth out of the water. It's important for birth attendants to be comfortable with many choices. There is no one way to have babies. If water is convenient and available, women should be as supported to birth there as anywhere else they might choose.

I think water and birth are becoming more and more popular because it's more of an ancient tradition than we know. With the introduction of the medicalization of childbirth, thousands of years of birth traditions were wiped out. We lost our great-grandmothers who passed down the knowledge of birth. This wisdom was turned into folktales and stories. This wisdom came to be considered witchcraft and not pertinent to medicine. The tradition of water, I think, is ancient and we're just rediscovering it. A midwife I met in Japan told me that many older midwives there have always used water in birth, perhaps for thousands of years. Now, in our society, we're giving ourselves the freedom to explore other modalities besides just the medical one and some of these ancient traditions are reappearing. We're reclaiming them.

I think the message in the fact that we're doing this, particularly with water birth, is freedom of choice and empowerment of women. Water heightens the awareness of consciousness and gives women the opportunity to be totally aware and present for this process of birth that confronts and transforms every fiber of a woman's being and every person's being that is involved. The water allows her to receive her baby consciously. Water is a graphic statement that birth can be achieved without the medical intervention that we have built up as the way to have a baby. Water gives women choices and allows them to follow their instincts.

An Imagined Baby's Perspective on Water and Bonding

by Rima Star

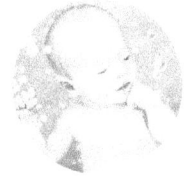

My mother labored in water and when she delivered me, she stepped outside the tub to the nearby grass patio. She squatted in the grass on a warm summer morning. The change from the water to outside the tub felt like a big downward sweeping of energy, helping me to move, and in moments, I was lying on the soft earth with my mother's warm hands picking me up and swooping me into her arms. I looked up into her face, surrounded by beautiful light, and was glad to be born. Soon after, my placenta—the pillow I had rested my head on—came out, we were both getting a little cool. She knew intuitively to return to the warm water. Moving from the patio to the tub with her holding me was a new experience, different from moving when I was inside the womb. It felt a little dangerous, even though I knew she would not drop me.

When she sat down in the tub and I felt the warm water all around me, I felt like I was smiling all over. This was home. How good I felt to be in this new place, but in a familiar water environment. I knew this was the big water my mother had been laboring in and bathing in before I was born. I had been wondering what it would feel like to be in the big water. Now I knew. It was terrific! What was especially terrific was to be held and floated in this womb water tub and be able to see my mother from the outside for the first time. She was gorgeous. More beautiful than I had possibly imagined. I felt like it was just her and me in a warm, supportive world. I was glad to be here. She was singing to me and smiling, welcoming me just as I was welcoming her.

I began to really be aware of my body and the fact that I could move my arms and legs, and really stretch them out without touching anything. I tried this stretching over and over again, and my mom would tell me what a big, wonderful world I had come into. I was feeling that she was right. It was different, but also exciting and pleasurable. One time, she drew me up towards her body and my feet pushed into her belly. That was strange but nice and soft—a little like pushing from the inside out.

I began to be aware of my mouth and tongue, and the desire to suckle. I opened and closed my mouth a few times, sticking my tongue out. No sooner had I done this than my mom floated me over to her body. My head turned automatically, and this warm, soft nipple was in my mouth. I began sucking and felt pleasure in this new activity. Soon, a liquid oozed out of the nipple and I swallowed it. It tasted good and felt warm inside my body. I relaxed and continued to suckle in the warmth of the tub, until I was full and dozing in the water. I was sure I had found Heaven on Earth. Soon, my mother took me from the tub and placed me in her bed next to her body and I slept for a long, long time.

In the days and weeks that followed, we had bath time every day, sometimes two or three times. I loved the water, and especially the undivided attention I received from my mother. Sometimes, she would hold me at the back of my neck, with my head upright, and I would feel like I could walk across the tub. Did I feel like a big person then! I also liked it when she held me on my stomach, and I could kick my legs and hands. I would splash water on me and her and we would laugh and laugh.

One time, she said to me, "You can still swim underwater just like when you were in the womb. You can hold your breath and I'll dip you under and up. Do you want to try it?" I said silently to her, "Yes, of course!" I had been wondering when she would think of this. She told me she was going to count to three, blow in my face, and dip me under. I did as she said and liked the game. It was fun to sail through the water with my head submerged. It seemed natural to me to hold my breath but a few times, I forgot and swallowed some water. It wasn't too bad. I sputtered and cleared my throat. I learned to pay close attention to when I was on top of the water and when I was going under. Eventually, I never missed holding my breath.

When I got bigger and she would swim me through the tub on my front, I would put my own head in and out of the water. When we got in our bigger hot tub, she and I would bob up and down together. I liked that because I could see her face underwater. There would be lots of bubbles and we would come up laughing. Sometimes, she would hold some colorful toy under the water, and I would try and grab it.

After we would play a while, she would float me over to her and I would nurse and fall asleep in the warmth of her arms. I felt so happy, strong, and grateful to be alive. Being in the water always made me feel that I could learn and do anything that I wanted to and that my mother truly cares for me.

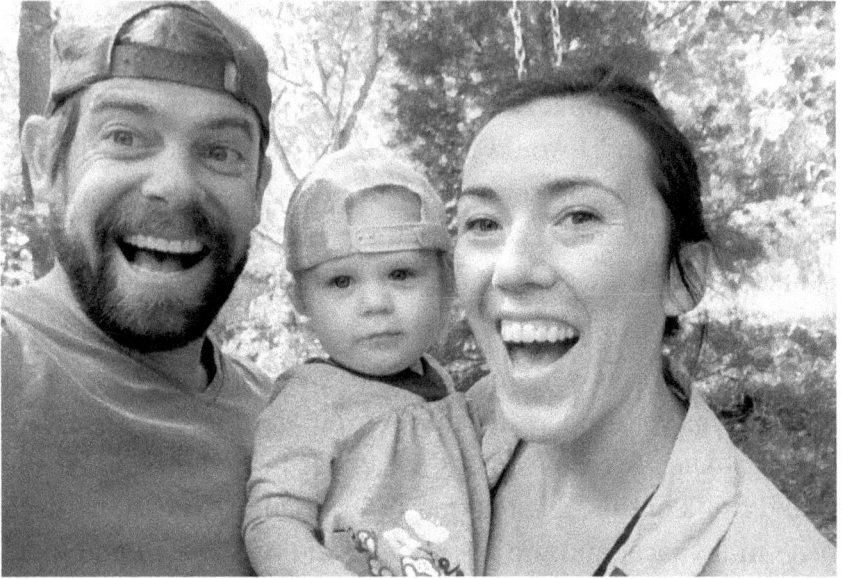

Figure 4.5. *Andy, Josie, and Orien celebrating their family life. Photo by Monet Nicole, used with permission.*

Endnotes

1   A. Merriam-Webster, *Ninth New Collegiate Dictionary*, Springfield, Massachusetts: Merriam-Webster Inc., 166.

2   Marshall H. Klaus MD. and John H. Kennell MD, *Bonding—The Beginnings of Parent-Infant Attachment*, St. Louis, Mo.,The C.V. Mosby Co., 1983, pp.1-2.

3   Klaus and Kennell, p.37

4   Klaus and Kennell, p.38

5   Klaus and Kennell, p.49

6   Klaus and Kennell, p.49

7   Klaus and Kennell, p.41

8   Klaus and Kennell, *Bonding*, p.56.

9   Cheyney, Melissa and Davis-Floyd, Robbie. "Birth and the Big Bad Wolf: Biocultural Evolution and Human Childbirth." In *Birthing Techno-Sapiens: Human-Technology Co-Evolution and the Future of Reproduction*, edited by Robbie Davis-Floyd. London, Routledge, pp. 15-46.

10   Gottlieb, Alma and De Loache, Judy. *A World of Babies: Imagined Childcare Guides for Eight Societies.* Cambridge University Press, 2017.

11   Klaus and Kennell, *Bonding*, p.4

12   Klaus and Kennell, *Bonding*, p.4-5.

13   Klaus and Kennell, *Bonding*, p.47

14   Odent, Michel, Unpublished Manuscript, 1990

15   Huxley, Laura Arachera, Piero Feruci, Illustrated by Paola Ferruci, *The Child of Your Dreams*, CompCare Publishers, Minneapolis, Minnesota, 1987, p.80.

16   Odent, Michel, *Water and Sexuality*, p.66.

17   Igor Charkovsky personal interview, Moscow, USSR, September, 1988. For an anthropological analysis and critique of Charkovsky's work, see Ozhiganova, Anna, "The Birth of a *New Human Being*: The Utopian Project of the Late Soviet Water Birth Movement and Its Inheritors." In *Birthing Techno-Sapiens: Human-Technology Co-Evolution and the Future of Reproduction*, edited by Robbie Davis-Floyd, 2021, pp. 193-207.

18   Odent, Michel, *Water and Sexuality*, p. 19-20.

19   See Davis-Floyd, Robbie and Elizabeth Davis, 2018. "Intuition as Authoritative Knowledge in Midwifery and Home Birth." *In Ways of Knowing about Birth: Mothers, Midwives, Medicine, and Birth Activism* by Robbie Davis-Floyd. Long Grove IL: Waveland Press, pp. 189-220.

20 Klaus, Marshall and Klaus, Phyllis, *The Amazing Newborn*, Addison-Wesley Publishing Co. 1985, p.7.

21 Klaus and Klaus, *The Amazing Newborn*, p. 96.

www.ingramcontent.com/pod-product-compliance
Lightning Source LLC
Chambersburg PA
CBHW062049270326
41931CB00013B/2997